D1198964

CLEAN EATING,

Dirty Sex

Sensual Superfoods and
Aphrodisiac Practices for Ultimate Sexual Health
and Connection

LISA DAVIS, MPH

RECIPES BY
ERIN MACDONALD, RDN

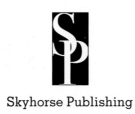

Skyhorse Publishing

Copyright © 2019 by Lisa Davis

All rights reserved. No part of this book may be reproduced in any manner without the express written consent of the publisher, except in the case of brief excerpts in critical reviews or articles. All inquiries should be addressed to Skyhorse Publishing, 307 West 36th Street, 11th Floor, New York, NY 10018.

Skyhorse Publishing books may be purchased in bulk at special discounts for sales promotion, corporate gifts, fund-raising, or educational purposes. Special editions can also be created to specifications. For details, contact the Special Sales Department, Skyhorse Publishing, 307 West 36th Street, 11th Floor, New York, NY 10018 or info@skyhorsepublishing.com.

Skyhorse® and Skyhorse Publishing® are registered trademarks of Skyhorse Publishing, Inc.®, a Delaware corporation.

Visit our website at www.skyhorsepublishing.com.

10 9 8 7 6 5 4 3 2 1

Library of Congress Cataloging-in-Publication Data

Names: Davis, Lisa.
Title: Clean eating, dirty sex: sensual superfoods and aphrodisiac practices
   for ultimate sexual health and connection / Lisa Davis, MPH ; recipes by
   Erin Macdonald, RDN.
Description: New York, NY: Skyhorse Publishing, [2018] | Includes index.
Identifiers: LCCN 2018040465| ISBN 9781510729988 (hardcover: alk. paper) |
   ISBN 9781510730007 (ebook)
Subjects: LCSH: Aphrodisiacs. | Sex (Biology)—Nutritional aspects. | Diet
   therapy.
Classification: LCC RM386 .D39 2018 | DDC 615.7/669—dc23 LC record available at https://lccn
   .loc.gov/2018040465

Cover design by Jenny Zemanek
Cover images courtesy of iStockphoto

Print ISBN: 978-1-5107-2998-8
Ebook ISBN: 978-1-5107-3000-7

Printed in China

DEDICATION

In memory of my mother. Thank you, Mom, for always believing in me and encouraging me to expand my horizons.

To my loving husband. I am blessed to share my life with you. Without your love and support, this book would not be possible. I appreciate all the sacrifices you have made, and continue to make, so I can make my dreams come true. I love you.

To my daughter. You are the light of my life. I love you.

In memory of Colleen, who believed in me before I ever did. I love you with all my heart.

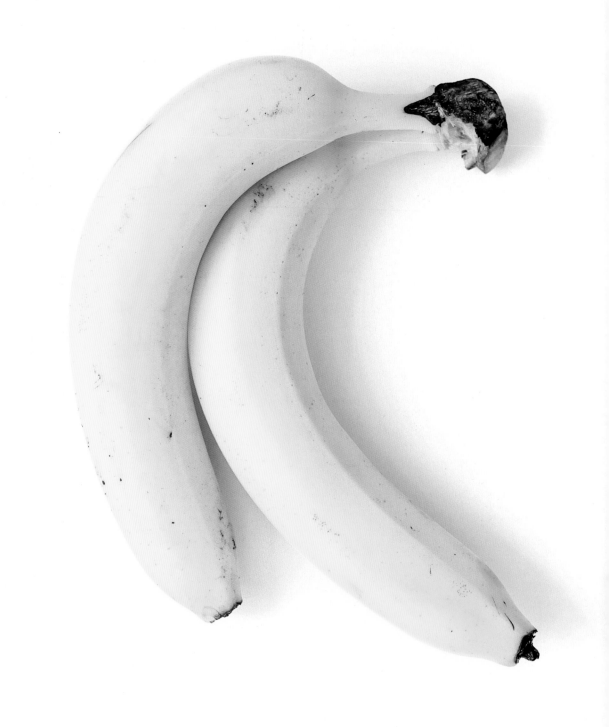

CONTENTS

FOREWORD BY JOE CROSS

I'm a logical guy and I like to think that I look at things in a logical way. And in my business world, I had become reasonably successful at solving problems. Only, over time, I eventually became the problem. My health failed me—or as it turns out, I failed my health. In solving my own health problems, I found I could do it without medication, and the unexpected benefit was I improved my sex life. Let me tell you the short version of my story.

I started out fit. But I was pretty much like any other regular American or Australian man. Busy, short on time, poor diet, and stressed out—stuck on the treadmill with nowhere to go, so to speak! At that point, it dawned on me that we are all jugglers. You can divide your life and everything that matters into five categories: Health, Career, Family/Friends, Love, and Self. And we are all trying to juggle these five buckets, if you like. That basically sums up being a human being in today's world. Now, I thought I was being smart when I decided it's easier to juggle two buckets than five. So, I put Health, Self, and Love aside, and decided to just focus on Family/Friends and Career.

Well, as you can imagine, that worked fine for a period of time. But in the long run it didn't work out too well. Sure, through the focus on my career, I accumulated more wealth, but at the direct expense of my health! I also enjoyed a party, so my friends and family got lots of "Joe Time." I wasn't a bad person, I was just not very kind to myself. My diet was very high in carbohydrates, fat, sugar, salt, and processed food. I also drank a lot of alcohol and soda, smoked a lot, and I didn't move much. I was someone who treated my body like a toxic waste dump. Sound familiar?

Pretty soon it became apparent that this lifestyle wasn't sustainable. My plan to juggle less by ignoring Health, Self, and Love came to a screeching end. I broke at age thirty-two and got Chronic Urticaria and Angioedema, a debilitating autoimmune disease affecting the skin. It wasn't just a case of taking a drug and I'd be fixed again. It was a sentence to medication for the rest of my life. Or so I was told!

I spent eight years taking medication, and hoping and praying I'd get better. I found out that the medications don't heal, they just suppress the symptoms. And because this was a disease of touch, my sex life suffered. While I never quite experienced erectile dysfunction (ED), I did experience low energy and a low sex drive. I suffered with a number of other debilitating symptoms due the autoimmune disease that made me very self-conscious, like welts on my skin and swelling in my joints!

At forty, I came to the realization I was responsible. Perhaps my lifestyle choices had something to do with it! I decided to take things in my own hands and instead of outsourcing my health to other people, pharmaceutical companies, and doctors—and trying all sorts of wacky and wonderful ideas—I came up with a plan to go on a plant-based diet.

I had one hundred pounds to lose, so I gave myself two years to reverse the effects of my previous lifestyle. I call this my "Reboot." I juiced just plants for sixty days, then I ate just plants for another three months. And to my surprise, I lost one hundred pounds, got off the medications, and got my health back. It didn't take two years like I thought—it took just five months. That was ten years ago and I'm still going strong. I now travel the world sharing my story in the hope that others can bring about positive changes to their life, just like I did.

And like Lisa, I found this worked for others, not just me. During my public events, the subject of sex is rarely raised, but I love to bring it up—it's a subject that will always get a few laughs. And as soon as you throw out the fact that, by default, when a man loses lots of belly fat, their appendage can appear bigger, you definitely know you have their attention! But seriously, once you start to discuss how blood flow and hormone balance can be affected by our diets, the audience is deathly quiet!

Apart from just feeling better about yourself and being more flexible, blood flow is a huge factor in that, if you clean out the system by getting rid of a substantial amount of processed foods that were making you sluggish and tired, and you replace that with mother nature's finest, you will decrease inflammation and by default increase blood flow and the capacity of your heart rate to sustain erections.

I've spoken to many men that are quite heavy, and it is very difficult for them to hold their bodies up with their arms. So, the only way they can have sex is on their side or on their back— which limits the sex positions open to them.

But as you get lighter, and you get your blood flowing more freely, it's about more than just being able to move. Your mental state becomes more confident and you are more confident about your body. All of those things parlay into a much more active, productive, and confident sex life. All of this is from the male side but of course for women, feeling confident and healthy in yourself physically and mentally is also equally rewarding.

I know Lisa from numerous visits on her radio shows and I know that her passion to help others live a healthier life in every area, not just in their sex lives, is real. In my travels, sharing my story, and on my website, I've seen people adopt Lisa's style of "clean eating," and change their lives. There's no reason you can't be one of them!

So, get into this book and take control, like I did. Let Lisa help you change your life with her practical advice in *Clean Eating, Dirty Sex*, and let's all rejoice by leaving the lights on a little more often!

Joe Cross,
Creator of the documentary "Fat, Sick & Nearly Dead," and author of *Juice It to Lose It, Reboot with Joe Juice Diet, 101 Smoothie Recipes*, and more
www.RebootWithJoe.com

INTRODUCTION

Hello, I'm Lisa Davis. During my twenty-plus years working in health education media, I have created television and radio programs to both educate and entertain. I believe learning is best accomplished with engagement and I find that both humor and relatable stories help the process.

It is my passion to inspire people to make healthy lifestyle changes and become the best versions of themselves. To that end, I have interviewed over 2,000 top experts in the field and presented our conversations in both audio and visual formats. Between their expertise and my educational and life experience, millions of listeners and viewers have come to trust the health information I dish out.

I seek out these experts to bring my listeners cutting-edge health advice. This format works so well for my popular podcasts and radio show that I used the same approach for this book. Included in these pages is the expertise from leading professionals in the fields of nutrition, lifestyle change, sex, and relationship. I know each expert from our prior interviews and they are the cashew-cream of the crop.

This book was conceived during a conversation with a friend. We were talking about my favorite health topics and the two areas in which I have experienced the most personal growth—food and sex.

Clean Eating, Dirty Sex: Sensual Superfoods and Aphrodisiac Practices for Ultimate Sexual Health and Connection is your guide to a healthier and sexier you. Filled with inspiring stories, science-based advice, and recipes, this hands-on book is designed to empower readers to make impactful lifestyle changes in the kitchen and the bedroom.

I stand by Hippocrates, the father of Western medicine, who said, "Let food be thy medicine and medicine be thy food." We know that we must eat to stay alive. But to nourish ourselves well is a crucial part to better physical and emotional health which will result in closer relationships with your partner and more fulfilling results between the sheets.

All of this implies change, which is not always easy. Fear not, for I shall share tips and tools on how to find your why, strengthen your resolve, and make lasting change. The advice that's given on every page of this book is designed to help you improve your health: physically, emotionally, and sexually.

The book follows the path from unhealthy eating habits (Part One) to a diet that will enhance all aspects of your life (Part Two); from sexual blocks (Part Three) to increased connection and sexual satisfaction (Part Four). Tips for stocking your pantry for pleasure (Part Five) are followed by a host of sensual and sexy recipes (Part Six).

The Reference Section (Part Seven) facilitates future learning with links to the generous and knowledgeable experts—please visit their websites for additional information and offerings.

Clean Eating, Dirty Sex, whether you read it as a healthy sex guide with recipes or use it as a cookbook loaded with extras, I wish for you the best of life's pleasures—in and out of the kitchen and bedroom.

Let's get cookin'!

Lisa Davis
Deep in eastern snow, 2018

Part One

DIRTY EATING: RECIPE FOR DISASTER

The roots deeply planted one hundred years ago, healthy eating has long been a part of my family tree. Convinced she survived the flu pandemic of 1918 because she had eaten all her vegetables while in the hospital, Grammy Em, my mom's mom, was our family's original health food nut. She passed her healthy culinary chops down to my mother, who in turn punished me.

The 1970s—bell bottoms, long hair, Saturday morning cartoons—for an elementary school-aged child in San Jose, California, life was good—until my mother started a new tradition. After enjoying cartoons (Schoolhouse Rock!), I *graciously* accepted my mother's *invitation* to accompany her to the local family-owned health food store.

Health food stores today are a cornucopia of organic multicolored maize, dark chocolate, colorful carbohydrates, international delicacies, fresh salad bars, hot and cold options ready to go—blending together into a medley of amazing aromas—a veritable feast for the senses. Back then . . . not so much. Our local store reeked of carob and cardboard, two of my least favorite snacks. Mom and I cruised the aisles for bulk millet, almonds, brown rice, bulgur wheat (more like *vulgar* wheat), carob, vitamins, and an array of other unappealing food-like items. What made the trip palatable was the small Tiger's Milk bar we shared. One. Singular. Uno. As a youth my mother was drafted into Grammy Em's Culinary Crusade—I chose to remain a cauliflower objector.

The commercial supermarket chain provided the bulk of our staples, and the occasional *junk food* treat: graham crackers, sans cinnamon-sugar topping, and Fig Newton's flavorless, drier cousin, Fig Bars.

Grown-ups' cookies. I vowed that when I grew up I would eat Cap'n Crunch cereal and children's cookies for dinner. I felt so deprived that I regularly raided the cupboards of my best friend's kitchen. Ferreting out any long-lost orphaned cookie or honey-coated nugget, no sugary confection could escape my deprived digits. My abilities did not go unnoticed by her older siblings, who dubbed me "Mini Mooch."

If finding junk food was my super power, my mother with her food-hiding powers was my arch nemesis. Once in a blue moon she would buy and then hide cookies, crackers, and my favorite at the time, Space Food Sticks (I envied the astronauts, floating in space, eating Space Food Sticks and drinking Tang). We knew she bought them, she didn't keep this a secret, but once she got them home it was "game on." When I was six, while jumping on my parents' bed, I spied the motherlode. It seemed a mirage. There they were, nestled on the highest shelf, beyond the reach of a child's outstretched arm—the elusive Space Food Sticks. Mustering all my strength and courage, I dragged a chair from the extra bedroom to the threshold of the closet. Needing more altitude, I stacked magazines atop the chair like a life-sized game of Blockhead (think colorful Jenga), and absconded with the goods before it all came tumbling down. I felt so guilty when my older, much taller brother got blamed, that I almost confessed—but like Daffy Duck, I was a "*gr-e-e-dy* little coward." Sorry, Bro!

Space Food Sticks got me through the lean times, but I craved something more. At nine the perfect opportunity fell into my lap—my Girl Scout Troop's annual cookie drive. Knowing that my mother would never allow me to buy "that junk," I sprung into action. I used months of saved allowance to order my allotment of cookies, all for myself! I cleared my green desk drawers of all important documents, and waited. And waited. Those drawers proved to be the perfect hiding place for my secret stash of Thin Mints.

My bad eating habits continued through my first three years of high school. I was super skinny (think "Olive Oyl," as the jocks in high school called me) and despite my best efforts, I never gained weight. As a last resort I increased my intake of junk food. The needle wouldn't budge. As a last, last resort I reluctantly went to the gym.

After my ten-minute workout—lift weights/check out guys (not necessarily in that order)—I headed outside for my run . . . to Taco Bell to get a beefy tostada with *no sour cream.* This seemed a very healthy choice to me and was definitely the highlight of my workout (well, that and the guys)! My *healthy* choices continued as I gained more independence, leaving the cocoon of cardboard and carob, and blazing my own SAD trail.

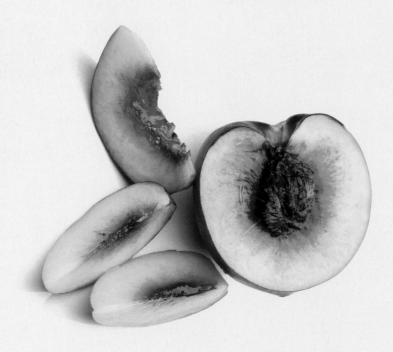

Chapter One

DIRTY DIETS ARE SAD

The Standard American Diet (SAD) is aptly named. The SAD diet consists of factory-farmed and processed meat, fried foods, fast food, frozen meals, refined grains, pizza, and high-sugar drinks. Michael Fenster, MD, author and integrative cardiologist, shared, "These foods are excessively high in added sugars and often rich in refined grains, carbohydrates, [bad] oils . . . and sorely lacking in fresh fruits and vegetables. This lack of balance results in some of the defining characteristics of the modern Western diet. It is energy dense but nutrient poor."

"Running on Empty" Is SAD

The hallmark of SAD foods is convenience and long shelf life. They are tailor-made for the *modern, go-go-go, no time to sit and enjoy a meal* lifestyle. This diet supplies short-term energy, creating cycles of sugar and carbohydrate highs and crashes. SAD eaters fill up on empty calories and do not get the essential nutrients their bodies need.

Dr. Fenster refers to the preponderance of foods that are highly processed, preserved, pre-prepared, and pre-packaged as the Four Horsemen of the Dietary Apocalypse. These SAD foods are the forerunners to diabetes, stroke, coronary artery disease, cancer, kidney and gallbladder disorders, hormone disruptions, inflammation, and a host of other physical and emotional conditions. It also kills your libido which results in a SAD sex life.

Addictive by Design Is SAD

I spoke with Pankaj Vij, MD, FACP, author of *Turbo Metabolism*, about the intentional manipulations by SAD food manufacturers. Dr. Vij shared:

> "You would think that there is some enemy who wants to take over America and they are feeding us this junk that is disguised as food. There are all these additives and poisons that are hiding that would slowly make us stupid, tired, and lazy so we cannot think for ourselves. However, the sad reality is that it is none of that. It is our own businesses; it is our food industry that is in cahoots with pharma industry and all they care about are profits. So they make these foods more tasty and addictive."
>
> "They use functional MRI machines with healthy volunteers to see which parts of their brains light up while they taste different flavors of their dressing, ketchup, sauce, or whatever seasoning that they are going to add. This way they can fine tune their products to make them hyper-palatable, leaving you wanting more. These are expensive pieces of equipment used in scientific research. These companies are so rich that they can invest in that type of technology.
>
> "We are surrounded by foods that are convenient, familiar, and hyper-palatable. They light up the reward centers of the brain like cocaine or heroin would. These people have no shame and they are proud of the fact that you cannot eat just one of their potato chips, ice cream, burgers, French fries or whatever it is. I would be the first to admit that it tastes

good. I grew up in another country and when I first came to America, my friend took me to a fast food place and I felt like my brain exploded with pleasure.

"These foods block your arteries, which can lead to things like high blood pressure, heart attack, or stroke. It is the same process that provides blood circulation to our sex organs. You can find erectile dysfunction if you are a man or lack of interest in sex if you are a woman. The same circulation provides blood flow to the brain. If you are not getting the fuel to the brain and you cannot think clearly, you can quickly develop things like Alzheimer's, memory loss, which as we are finding is all related to metabolism. These are metabolic diseases. We have so called chronic disease, which fill up doctors' offices every day and are totally preventable. 80% of the cure is in food."

Sugar Is Not a Food Group—It's SAD

Michael Klaper, MD, is a world-renowned physician, consultant, and educator who specializes in plant-based nutrition. Dr. Klaper advises to avoid alcohol, fried foods, simple carbohydrates, and refined sugars such as candy, table sugar, syrups, and soft drinks.

We spoke about the dangers of processed sugar. Dr. Klaper explained, "Manufacturers extract the sugar from sugar beans and sugar cane and turn it into refined white sugar. Corn syrup is made into high fructose corn syrup. The modified molecules from sugar production are trouble makers that damage our bodies in a number of ways.

"When you eat a candy bar, or drink a cola drink, you flood your tissues with sugar and these sugar molecules lock onto your protein. The sugar-protein combination is a destructive end product that damages every tissue in the body. For example, it damages the clear protein in your eyes—setting people up for cataracts. It damages the lining of the capillaries where oxygen gets into our tissues and as a consequence, ages the tissues and ages skin. Sugar creates inflammation," Dr. Klaper told me. Inflamed capillaries reduce blood flow to sexual organs, impacting libido and performance in bed.

Dr. Klaper remarked that modified carbohydrates were never meant to be eaten as a food. "You can get away with a little, like a half a teaspoon of maple syrup in your tea; but when you're eating a piece of coffee cake, or a muffin or donut or a candy bar, you're eating a chunk of sugar and the volume floods your tissues and causes a lot of damage to your body." He talked about certain food vendors like they're selling poison. Dr. Klaper warns, "If you walk into a bakery, be aware they are selling sugar in there, and while it looks and smells great, it's not going to help you meet your goals for sexual health."

Fats: The Good, the Bad, and the Oily

Here is the skinny on fats. For years fats were demonized (remember Snackwells?). People were buying low-fat this and low-fat that, not realizing the essential role healthy fats play in their diet.

The Good

Fats. Gotta love 'em! Well, the good ones. Steven Masley, MD, nutritionist, chef, author, and the creator of *30 Days to a Younger Heart* on PBS, dubbed the following "Smart Fats." These fats increase blood flow and regulate the production of sex hormones. Most of these oils and all of the foods on the following list contain omega-3 fatty acids.

Oils	Food Sources
almond oil	avocados
avocado oil	coconuts
extra-virgin olive oil	dark chocolate
fish oil	nuts (preferably raw)
hazelnut oil	olives
virgin coconut oil	wild salmon

The Bad

I watched a lot of television growing up and I clearly remember commercials for Wesson Oil (always loved Florence Henderson aka "Carol Brady"), Chiffon ("It's not nice to fool Mother Nature"), and who can forget Crisco ("You can trust Crisco Oil to fry chicken that doesn't taste greasy") extolling the virtues of vegetable oils.

I spoke with Lori Shemek, PhD, CNC, author of *How to Fight FATflammation!*, *Lasting Weight Loss,* and *Fire-Up Your Fat Burn!* Dr. Shemek said, "These unhealthy cooking oils (canola, corn, cottonseed, peanut, safflower, soybean, and 'vegetable oil') are clear, tasteless, highly refined, and processed. They are very high in omega-6 fat resulting in inflammation and leaving us fat and sick with diseases ranging from heart disease to obesity to cancer.

"Ideally, we need a 1:1 balance of omega-3 to omega-6. Right now, that balance is 1:28 in favor of omega-6. When we have too much of an omega-6 fat intake, omega-3 cannot adequately do its job of reversing inflammation. Adding more omega-3 fat should be a priority for all." With inflammation comes poor blood flow, a lowered libido, and a lackluster performance in bed.

The Oily: Good Fats Gone Bad

Sometimes, even *good* cooking oils can turn *bad*. According to Dr. Masley, "Typically around 350° Fahrenheit, chemical compounds in the oils break down and become oxidized. This is particularly true of delicate oils that have a lot of flavor, like extra-virgin olive oil, coconut oil, and sesame oil. Using coconut oil for high heat cooking is a huge myth."

I recommend doing your high heat cooking with oils that can withstand the high temperatures, such as avocado oil, almond oil, and hazelnut oil. Avocado oil is my go-to and I always use Avohass. Not only does it have a high smoke point (520°F), I think it's delicious!

Each oil has a slightly different flavor, which can bring depth to your meals. The important thing to keep in mind is to use these oils in their natural, unrefined state. Dr. Masley adds, "If you really love the flavor of coconut oil, olive oil, or sesame, you could always add a little to your food once it is cooked."

Chapter Two

DIRTY FOODS:
THE FAST LANE TO CRASHING HEALTH

Drew's Story: From Fit to Fat to Fit

Drew Manning, a bodybuilder, fitness coach, and owner of *www.Fit2Fat2Fit.com*, would often hear from his frustrated clients, "Drew, you don't understand how hard this is. You've never had to struggle the way I do!" In an effort to better relate to his clients, Drew cooked up a plan. He would walk in his clients' shoes—as little as possible.

A Flabulous Plan

Drew decided to get fat on purpose. For six months, he didn't exercise and ate the Standard American Diet. He consumed ready-to-eat cereals, white breads, granola bars, crackers, cookies, macaroni and cheese, frozen foods, sugary juices, soft drinks, and fast food. His food choices were based on convenience, not health, and consisted of highly processed, preserved, pre-prepared, and pre-packaged foods.

"I just ate whatever I wanted," Drew said. Unlike the typical standard American diet, he ate only when hungry and limited his intake of fast food to twice a week.

Drew gained seventy-six pounds in six months. The weight gain affected every area of his life, especially his sex life. Drew experienced loss in libido, decreased self-esteem, sleep loss, and mood and personality changes.

Although Drew anticipated the physical changes, he was humbled by the mental and emotional effects he had not expected. He experienced bouts of sadness and apathy, became

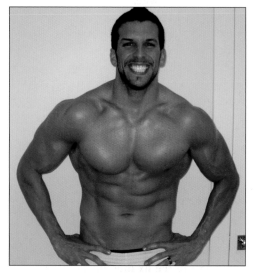

Drew in 2011 before he gained weight.

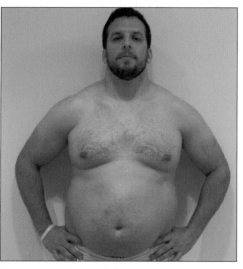

Drew seventy-six pounds heavier . . .

lazy, stopped helping around the house and with the kids, and started complaining constantly. He had a two-year-old daughter at the time and there was a moment when she started crying because he could no longer keep up with her. His change in mood and attitude caused friction with his wife.

"I lost my identity, in a way. My self-esteem was low; I didn't want to see myself naked and turned the lights off to be intimate with my wife and even avoided her when I came out of the shower. I started snoring pretty quickly upon gaining weight and could no longer reach those deep stages of sleep. My hormones got off which affected my mood and my personality." Drew was glad he stopped after six months, "It was kind of a dangerous slippery slope."

Here are Drew's photos, before he gained weight, and two photos after six months of SAD eating and no exercise.

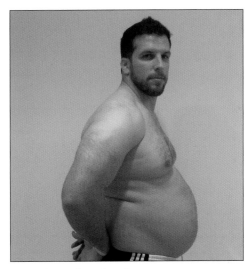

. . . and view from the side.

A Flab-U-Loss Plan

At the end of the six months, Drew took measured steps as he shifted back to his previous lifestyle. In month one, he changed his diet. In month two, he gradually added exercise until he built back up to his previous workout routine.

The most surprising aspect of losing the weight was the long plateaus during which the scale refused to budge. Despite his disciplined efforts to do everything *right*, there were times, for a week or two, or sometimes longer, when he didn't lose a pound. He recalled his clients' results had flatlined even when they followed the personalized plan he made for them. It took Drew six months to lose the seventy-six pounds and get back to where he was before.

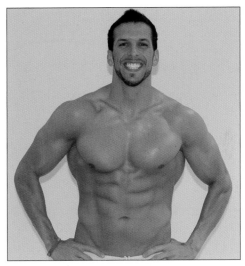

Drew after he gained and then lost weight.

Andrea's Story: The Power of Knowledge

Andrea Donsky, nutritionist and health media expert, was not always savvy about her diet. She was brought up on healthy food but when she was a teenager she started eating and drinking unhealthy fast food, candy, and soda. After she left home and her mother's healthy cooking behind, she continued to eat junk foods and experienced bloating and gas each time she ate.

Motivated by digestive problems and wanting to understand the root causes, Andrea researched and discovered that her symptoms were a direct result of her food choices. Once she understood nutrition, she started to listen to her body. If a food made her feel bloated or sluggish, she would remove this food and replace it with a healthy alternative. She lost weight, increased energy, eliminated the gas and bloating, and felt amazing.

Her growing knowledge and interest in diet and her transformational experience prompted her to return to school to become a holistic nutritionist. "The biggest tip I have for anyone trying to live a healthier lifestyle is, 'Listen to your body.' Our bodies know exactly what we do and don't want and what it does and doesn't need."

Genetic Testing

Andrea recently had genetic testing done. "Genetic testing takes the guesswork out for you. It prevents the trial and error of having to try many different diets. It opened up my world for me." With an at-home kit from a company called Youtrients, Andrea discovered that her body can't digest starch. "I went Paleo and lost nine pounds within three weeks." Genetic testing may help you discover to which foods you may be particularly sensitive.

The Scary 7

Her book *Unjunk Your Junk Food* was a response to the typical kid-oriented SAD foods her toddlers were served at so many birthday parties and playdates. Andrea shared her list of "The Scary 7" ingredients to look for and *avoid*.

1. High fructose corn syrup
2. Trans fat, shortening, hydrogenated (or partially-hydrogenated) glycerides (mono- & di-)
3. "Artificial flavors" (blanket term for over one hundred possible chemical additives)
4. Monosodium glutamate (MSG)
5. Artificial colors
6. Artificial sweeteners (aspartame, sucralose, acesulfame potassium (ACE-K), neotame, and saccharin)
7. Preservatives (TBHQ, polysorbates, BHT/BHA, nitrates, nitrites, potassium sorbate, sodium benzoate, and sulfides)

For optimal health, read food labels. Andrea adds, "Read the ingredients and not just the nutrition facts panels. The ingredients tell the whole story. Don't rely on front-of-package labeling or claims. Make sure to understand what you're reading. If the list of ingredients is long and complicated, put the product back on the shelf and lastly, avoid "The Scary 7"—download the full list and take it shopping with you."

Charles's Story: It Takes a Village

Celebrity chef Charles Mattocks, also known as *The Poor Chef*, is a bestselling author, and has made multiple television appearances on *The Today Show*, *Good Morning America*, *Fox News*, *The Talk*, *Martha Stewart*, CBS TV, CNN, and *Dr. Oz*.

Inspired by his uncle, the late reggae legend Bob Marley, Charles dared to dream big! After being diagnosed with diabetes in 2011, Charles set out on a global mission to save not only his life, but also millions with diabetes with his reality TV show, *Reversed*.

Reversed follows the lives of individuals affected by diabetes. While the camera is rolling, courageous participants share their struggles to change their diet, fitness, and mentality in order to control and reverse their diabetes.

Charles told me, "*Reversed* was born out of the need to inspire and educate millions. Participants and viewers learn how to change the way they eat, drink, think, exercise, and live with diabetes. With over 380 million worldwide plagued with diabetes, thirty-five million in America alone and counting, 189 million walking around that don't know they have diabetes—we have a pandemic on our hands."

In 2018, I joined Charles's "Diabetes Dream Team" for the second season of *Reversed*. It's a dream come true to work alongside so many dedicated people including Ward Bond, PhD; Beth Frates, MD; Michael Fenster, MD; and Lori Shemek, PhD, who are also featured in this book.

Diabetes

Diabetes is a serious disease that can have major consequences if not properly treated. With Type 2 diabetes, your body has trouble using or making enough insulin. Insulin is a hormone that helps the sugar from your food enter your cells to be used for energy. If the sugar cannot enter the cells it builds up in the blood stream causing high blood sugar. The most frequent health problems associated with poorly controlled blood sugar include heart disease, kidney disease, neuropathy (nerve damage in extremities) which can lead to amputations, and eye diseases such as glaucoma and cataracts. What most doctors don't tell you is that diabetes impacts your libido and blood flow to your sexual organs. Erectile dysfunction and inability to achieve an orgasm are very common and can be prevented.

The Poor Chef

Charles shared the following story with me on my podcast, *Talk Healthy Today*.

"About eight years ago I was diagnosed with diabetes and it was a shock! It was ironic because I was making my name as a celebrity chef, cooking healthy meals for cost effective prices. My book was *Eat Cheap but Eat Well*.

"I started getting some symptoms, specifically urinary frequency. I'd had it before and I usually went to a local Saturday clinic. I'd walk out the door with some antibiotics. One time a doctor asked if I had a family history of diabetes and I thought, 'What? Diabetes!' As a black male in his thirties who doesn't know anything about diabetes, I was terrified. The doctor at the clinic did a finger prick test; I had just eaten a large lunch. The doctor said he can put me on some medication and I thought, *Whoa. I need to see my regular doctor.*

"Once I saw my doctor and was told I did have diabetes, I thought about what I needed to do. I worked out with weights in the gym but I needed to add some cardio. I needed to get educated.

"As I started to research I began understanding the landscape of diabetes and the business of diabetes. I learned about the issues, complications, and the lack of education a person receives when they are diagnosed. Seeing this lack of education and the immense complications from this disease started my diabetes mission."

Reversed

"People need to make changes to slow down the devastation that diabetes has on the entire body. In order to do that you must know what diabetes is. You have to read, you have to study, you have to understand how foods work in your body, that proper sleep is key, and the impact of stress. When I was diagnosed I was working like a dog, wasn't exercising that much, and was stressed. Those were all contributing factors to the diabetes.

"With diabetes a lot of us gets the medication and just go home. We don't get the education. We need to take it upon ourselves to learn. This is one of the reasons why I created the television show *Reversed*. We need education that is engaging and informative. Where people watching can feel supported and feel less alone. There are so many different ways that you can combat this condition, including reading this book."

Part Two

CLEAN EATING:
HIGHWAY TO HEALTH

For most of my public primary education, fear of failure was queen. I quit everything because of her—quitting was my primary source of aerobic activity.

First grade was the first time I was picked last for a team—it would not be the last. After everyone else was picked, I was left standing while the teams argued about who would *get stuck* with me—this continued until high school.

Second grade was the first time I let fear decide my fate. I quit tap dancing to avoid the recital performance. This was difficult because I was jealous of my best friend who continued without me and especially envious of her sparkly recital outfits.

My lack of confidence was exacerbated due to my fear of PE (Physical Education). I thought of it then as Predictable Embarrassment. The last straw was sixth grade soccer. Years of humiliation had taught me—*walk, run, skip, crawl, burrow*—avoid the ball, avoid the taunts, avoid the pain. I swear, I was minding my own business, trying to remain invisible in the corner of the field—when it happened. That rotten ball found me.

I did not want to kick it. I wished someone would take it away. Where was Linus's sister Lucy when you needed her?! I stuck my foot out and pushed it away. I liked how it felt. I stepped up and kicked it. Then I followed that ball, running and kicking, kicking and running. To my surprise and joy, my feet maintained control of the ball. I was exhilarated. I dribbled that ball up the field. I was a natural. The other kids were actually calling out, "Go Lisa!" It was a refreshing change of pace from, "Come on! Don't just stand there!"

For the first time, I was excited about PE and school. The next day when PE was announced, I uncharacteristically *ran* to the field *with* my classmates. This was going to be great! Mr. Pederson reached into the PE bag and pulled out a baseball and bat—my heart sank. No more soccer?! In that moment, I learned an important life lesson: *Always give up, Always surrender!* In retrospect, I spent so much time being afraid of trying that I lost an amazing opportunity; unfortunately, it would not be the last time.

Junior high school provided a temporary reprieve, until the new kids realized they didn't want me on their team. By high school, the combination of being picked last, feeling like a loser, and being let down the one time I believed I could succeed had left me without the will to ever try again.

My mother begrudgingly allowed me to quit dance, band, tennis, *tree climbing*, and other activities, always cautioning, "You'll be sorry when you're older."

Surrendering was always an option—until yoga. My mother refused to let me quit. I wanted to put my foot down but it was already inching its way up the wall. No surrendering. I was going to do yoga.

Being forced to do yoga was the start of getting ready, to be ready, to change. It was also the start of taking my mother's health advice seriously. Yoga was the recommended remedy for my mild scoliosis. I had no other choice than to fully dedicate myself to the painful practice. Health and functioning were critically important to my mother.

My mom had three unsuccessful knee surgeries, which left her in chronic pain. She said she felt trapped in her body, unable to play tennis or comfortably carry out daily chores. Ice was her constant companion; she brought it with her everywhere she went. When I was in eighth grade, my mother developed an autoimmune illness that covered her in rashes and left her emaciated. It was heartbreaking. She continued to be ill for years without any answers.

When my interest in yoga waned, my mom encouraged me to try lap swimming. It was a natural fit—some of my fondest childhood memories are goofing around in the tennis club pool with my family. It seemed a good way to recapture happy times and follow in my mother's flippers. My first time lap swimming—the buoyancy of the water, my entire body in coordinated movement, nothing and no one to distract me—awakened within me the desire to make lasting change. Soon I was doing regular workouts in the pool and it was adios Taco Bell.

Was it easy to say goodbye to my beefy tostada with *no sour cream*? Heck no! My drive to be healthy outweighed, and eventually outlasted, my cravings.

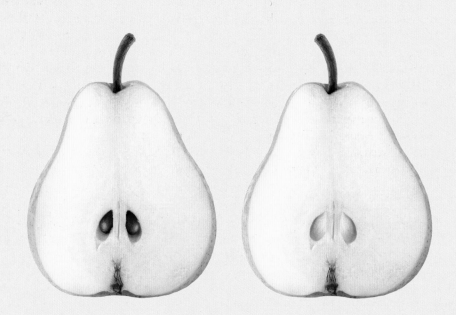

Chapter Three

BE THE CHANGE: DEFINE YOUR LIFESTYLE

W e have arrived at an exciting juncture, the place where *the shopping cart wheels meet the clean-food aisle floors*. I'll save the bootcamp-style pep talk for someone else and simply put you on notice that you will need to get up out of your comfy reading position, because I have a "To Do" list for you! All of the following advice and information is key to improving your health, your relationship with yourself and your partner, and ultimately, your time in the bedroom.

Diet, Not Dieting

I make the distinction between what we eat (diet) and a restrictive eating style designed for weight loss (dieting). Most people gain additional weight as a result of dieting because they unintentionally put their body into starvation mode. In starvation mode, all internal processes slow down to conserve energy because the body is not getting enough fuel. This creates sluggishness and sugar cravings, leading people to grab quick sugary or salty snacks in an attempt to replenish their depleted energy stores. The end product of dieting is long-term weight gain and chronic yo-yo dieting which may cause serious health problems and frustration rather than lasting change.

Dieting and SAD diets also affect the production of sex hormones, resulting in lowered libido, reduced blood flow, and an inability to achieve the heights of pleasure with your partner. Changing what you eat and your relationship with food takes work. You have to look deep within yourself to understand the "why" behind food choices, food restriction, or overconsumption, and reasons for eating that have nothing to do with physical hunger.

The following sections will help you to uncover your "why," which will allow you to make successful lifestyle changes that will result in better physical, emotional, and sexual health.

The *Bon Vivant* Girl

Bon Vivant is French for "Living Well" and the motto of Nathalie Botros, certified health coach and author of *If You Are What You Eat, Should I Eat a Skinny Girl?* Before arriving at a place of self-acceptance and healthy eating, Nathalie tried hundreds of diets. "Name the diet and I've tried it. Low-carb, high-protein, South Beach, holistic, vegetarian, rice, juicing." She's tried diet pills, acupuncture, liposuction, and even injected herself with pregnancy hormones in an effort to produce the desired dress size or number on the scale.

Some of those diets helped her lose weight, temporarily. As soon as she finished the diet, she said she felt invincible and started to fall back on former eating habits. "No surprise, I gained back the weight and even added a few more pounds." Nothing had changed, I just put my body into restriction and then into indulgence.

Nathalie shared, "I was a serial dieter and I was restricting myself from living. When I came to this conclusion, I decided no more diets for me. I needed a new lifestyle." It took her some time to get there. "During that period, I had highs and lows with my weight. This time, I didn't panic when I gained a few pounds. Instead, I had to study myself. The key was to understand why I gained that weight. Was it emotional or simply a hungry period? Studying my weight gain helped me to resolve that issue."

Tips for Living Well

Here are healthy practices that are within your reach. Nathalie shared sound advice that worked for her:

- Keep a food journal
- Don't keep junk food in your house
- Read the nutritional labels on your food
- Don't buy the hundred-calorie snack packs (highly processed junk)
- Eat real, whole foods
- Get a high-speed blender
- Sit down at a table and eat without distractions (no smartphone)
- Slow down and savor your meal, chew slowly, and pause between mouthfuls

Adopting New Habits: Are We There Yet?

The common notion that it takes twenty-one days to form a new habit is actually a modern myth with an interesting history. In 1960, plastic surgeon Dr. Maxwell Maltz observed his patients and deduced that it takes a *minimum* of twenty-one days to form a new habit.

Dr. Lori Shemek said, "New research shows it takes sixty-six days." In the habit study published in 2009, the average length of time was sixty-six days; the range was eighteen days to 254 days, depending upon the behavior.

Dr. Shemek advocates what I'm encouraging you to do here—take small, consistent steps in the direction you want to go and keep at it even if it looks like your results stall for a while. Be patient and stay the course.

"Like a Rolling Stone"

Inspired by the proverb, "A rolling stone gathers no moss," Beth Frates, MD, lifestyle medicine specialist, health and wellness coach, and the founder of Wellness Synergy LLC, developed a goal-setting method she calls MOSS: Motivators, Obstacles, Strategies, and Strengths™. "Just like the rolling stone, if you keep moving, moss cannot grow on you or in you," Dr. Frates told me. "Adopting new habits takes time. You need patience. You also need a plan."

Dr. Frates continued:

In order to keep the stone rolling, we need to keep creating goals and keep working towards our optimal state of wellness by eating healthy foods, exercising, sleeping, and using stress resiliency techniques.

Before tackling the MOSS in your life, it is important to craft a vision of yourself, not only in the immediate and shorter range goals of clean eating and increased pleasure, but in five years, ten years, or even twenty years. By creating a vision, you set a target. Ask yourself, "How will I be talking and walking? What activities will I be doing? Who will I be spending time with?" Envision yourself doing something you enjoy and use all your senses to describe it—sights, sounds, smells, tastes, and textures. The more concrete, the better. If you want, draw it or make a collage.

After you have completed work on your vision, you are ready to figure out how you will get there. You might need to adopt new healthy habits and maintain other ones in order to reach your vision.

Motivation

Dr. Frates continued, "Identifying compelling motivators is key. What is your motivation for changing certain behaviors? Why do you want to be like this in one, five, ten, or more years? It is essential to identify a compelling motivator that speaks to you when you are trying to adopt a new healthy behavior."

Find Your Why

As a health and lifestyle coach, I would go into people's homes, clean out their cupboards, take them shopping, and teach them how to prepare healthy meals. Before we started we would sit at their kitchen table and I would ask them to *find their why*. Without them understanding their why, knowing their why, what we did was less likely to stick.

Dr. Vij agrees,

I think the biggest piece is the "why." You start with the why because once you have a strong why for whatever it is that you are trying to do, the where, who, how, and when would all fall into place. You have to peel the onion a few times and really ask why five or six times. Why do I want this? Why do I really want this? Why am I really doing this?

Let us get to the bottom of the real motivation. The real thing that motivates me is my lifetime dream of climbing Mount Everest or my dream of being able to play tennis with my grandson and beat him in one game. To me, those are bigger goals than just looking good in a dress.

Finding out what that why is and when we peel the different layers of the onion, we find out that we are all very similar. We all like to have beautiful experiences. We all like to learn new things. We all like to grow and contribute in some way. Those are our highest needs and those cannot be fulfilled if we do not have good energy flow and we are tired and foggy-headed all the time.

Obstacles

Once you have a vision and you defined your why, Dr. Frates continued:

Next, think about what will get it your way. Once obstacles are identified, they can be managed. What will stop you from fulfilling that vision or from meeting your goals? Brainstorm about what could go wrong or things already in place that seem to be stumbling blocks.

Common obstacles include not having enough time to devote to adopting a new healthy habit, feeling comfortable with the current routine even though it is leading you down an unhealthy path, a spouse who practices unhealthy habits, demanding hours at work, and family problems or issue with children. All of these obstacles are challenging, but they are not impossible to surpass.

Strategies

Spend time strategizing ways around the obstacles you identified. The more solutions you think of, the more likely you will find a viable one. Finding solutions will increase your confidence that you can meet your goals and succeed in living your vision. Sometimes brainstorming with a friend can help you to be inventive and creative.

Strengths

Uncovering your strengths, gifts, and talents will empower you to tackle the obstacles and to persevere through the process. If you can't think of any of your strengths on your own, ask someone close to you. Speaking about our own strengths is not always comfortable for us. However, it is important to acknowledge your gifts and talents so that you can set yourself up for success in the long run. Everyone is unique, and everyone has strengths. To be our best, we need to use our strengths as often as possible.

Keep the Change

"Mindset is everything. It is important to think of everything in terms of lifestyle, health, and well-being. Our thoughts, words, and actions are powerful and we influence our ability to make long lasting change and to thrive from a mind/body perspective," said Denise McDermott, MD, a board-certified adult and child psychiatrist specializing in an integrative approach to mental health.

Dr. Denise gives the following advice to her patients for creating their Integrative Well-Being plans.

Write it down and be specific. Think of it as your unique health manifestation plan. Be realistic. If you have not been exercising for a while, do not start with forty-five- to sixty-minute cardio workouts. Start at your own pace and keep track of your own personal wins.

Keep it simple. Make one change at a time. One of my patients needed to *kick soda to the curb* to reduce her sugar intake. She made this one change and was able to lose inches around her waist and feel more energized.

Involve loved ones. It is amazing when we find a close friend or family member to start a new routine with whether it is with nutrition or fitness. Having a household that integrates healthy habits for everyone helps all of us to stay on track.

Be kind to yourself. Remember you are supposed to have fun while striving for health. If you miss a workout or eat a sugar snack, get right back on track and don't punish yourself!

Stay in a space of gratitude. I like to start my day thinking of what I am grateful for. This helps all of us to start from a positive mindset and helps us to make healthy choices.

Practice mindfulness. What does this mean? It means being in this moment, the "NOW." Having a non-judgmental view and observation of our behavior allows for self-awareness. This has a "ripple effect" of mind, body, soul alignment.

Don't forget to laugh! Laughter is the best medicine. We are supposed to have fun while staying healthy!

Sexy Together

Making changes together can be supportive and fun. No matter your current lifestyle and satisfaction in the kitchen and bedroom, no starting point is too low and no step is too small. Starting with even five minutes of movement, eliminating drinking sodas, and adding a salad every day, every small success is a win!

If you and your partner are super motivated, you can change your diet overnight. Otherwise, I suggest you take it easy and introduce one or two good foods at a time, increase your movement, and start drinking water.

Ideally, you and your partner will benefit the most from clean eating all day, every day. This doesn't have to be all or nothing to work. Allow yourself a few treats and you'll be ahead of the health curve if at least 80% of your diet is clean.

Have fun with it, cook together, and discuss the healthy changes you are experiencing. Keep in mind that you are doing this to improve your own health as well as your love life.

Smooth It Over

If you think your partner may balk at switching from junk food to clean food, but is open to surprise, I suggest you make a smoothie and invite your partner to chat.

Smoothies are an exceptionally easy and surprisingly tasty way to prepare clean food in less than ten minutes. So take advantage of that. If your partner shows resistance, let them know the creamy and tasty beverage they are enjoying contains clean ingredients. You'll be on the path to change! For ideas, check out Chapter Twenty, Sensual Smoothies and Milkshakes (page 167).

A Little Help from a Friend

I met Paul when he came to stay with our mutual friend Betty, a long-time clean eater. Paul was surprised to discover that although they were both sixty years old, Betty did not suffer from back pain, obesity, and mobility issues as he did. Paul asked if she would share her secret to maintaining her health. Betty offered to show him.

Betty doubled her shopping list and packed him five days of healthy food in separate bags and put it in the refrigerator on Sunday night. He didn't have to stop eating what he liked, he just had to promise to eat what she prepared.

For the next three months, Paul's breakfast consisted of a cup of heated bone broth, two hard-cooked eggs and a small container of "light" (low sugar) probiotic yogurt. For the rest of the day, he ate the variety of healthy items in the prepared bags. The contents changed with the seasons, but always contained a handful of almonds, a handful of walnuts, an apple, and two or three other seasonal fruits and vegetables.

Within a month he was finding that he needed less food to become full and asked Betty to please put less food in the bags. As he increased his intake of healthy foods, his appetite for fast food waned and he craved it less.

He continued to adjust his eating routine while at his beach house on weekends, even becoming a regular at the local juice bar. He especially enjoyed the spinach, kale, apple, and banana smoothie.

By the end of three months, Paul shed twenty-six pounds and felt great. Both his confidence and sleep improved. His newly increased energy and focus improved his work habits and efficiency. He expanded his business, improved his social life, and is eternally grateful to Betty.

Chapter Four

SUPERFOODS FOR A SUPERYOU

Betty, who we met at the close of Chapter Three, planned, shopped, and prepared three months of healthy food for Paul. If you are like me, and you do not have a *Betty* in your life, I encourage you to try on the new slogan, "Be Your Own Betty" (BYOB). To BYOB, use the list of clean ingredients in this chapter to boost your clean-eating quotient. Add these essential superfoods to your diet by making fabulous meals from the recipes in this book.

Water

My love of water goes beyond swimming. I drink a glass of water first thing every morning to hydrate my cells, during and after a hearty walk with the dogs, and throughout the day, even if I don't feel thirsty. A piece of good news from the habit study: Adding a daily glass of water took only eighteen days to become a habit!

Dr. Shemek told me that consuming sodas, other sugar-filled beverages, salty foods, and alcohol leads to dehydration. To avoid being left high and dry, always carry water with you in either a steel, non-BPA plastic, or lead-free glass bottle.

The Taste of Water

Many people avoid drinking water because they don't like the taste of water in general, or they don't like the chlorine taste of tap water. According to Joy Wildflower, PE, drinking water engineer, a simple carbon filter, in a pitcher or attached to your faucet, will remove chlorine from tap water. Ms. Wildflower suggests, "Change your filter according to the manufacturer's recommended frequency. Ask your water provider for information about the source and water quality of what comes through your faucet. Most public tap water is pure, wholesome, and potable. So I encourage everyone to take it from the tap!"

To enhance the flavor of water, Dr. Shemek suggests to pour yourself a tall glass of water and add fruit directly or with an infuser water bottle designed for this purpose. Slices of lemon, lime, orange, cucumber, and watermelon, or herbs like spearmint and basil, not only add flavor, they make for an attractive, fun, and healthy hydrating experience. I encourage you to try combinations, like adding basil with fruit or make your own lemon-lime!

Beneficial Bacteria

The human gut is teeming with trillions of colonies of bacteria; some are beneficial friends that keep us healthy and happy, while others are fearsome foes which undermine our health. Improve your gut microbiome by increasing the diversity and strength of the good bacteria and killing off the bad guys.

Adding friendly bacteria to your diet by eating fermented foods (like kimchi, kombucha, and sauerkraut), prebiotic foods (such as asparagus, dark chocolate, garlic, jicama, and onions), probiotic-rich foods (kefir, low-sodium miso, plain yogurt, and unfiltered apple cider vinegar, for example), digestive enzymes found in grains and sprouted breads, and omega-3 rich foods (chia seeds, dark leafy greens, ground flax seeds, walnuts, and wild salmon) will do wonders for a healthier gut.

Flavonoids

Flavonoids have strong antioxidant properties that increase blood vessel strength and blood flow throughout your body, and most notably to your sexual organs. This increased circulation not only increases arousal, it is also essential to avoid heart attacks in both men and women. This is why cardiovascular health is important for everyone.

Flavonoids contribute to the vibrant colors of fruits and can be found in nuts, seeds, grains, berries (especially blueberries), red wine, apples, dark chocolate, beans, lentils, and tea. This is why my mother told me to eat the peels on fruits and the white stringy, spongy substance (pith) between the orange flesh and the peel—they are loaded with flavonoids.

Good "Healthy" Fats

My radio family knows I champion healthy fats. Another advocate of healthy fats is Dave Asprey, founder of *Bulletproof*, creator of *Bulletproof Coffee*, host of the #1 health podcast, "Bulletproof Radio," and author of the *New York Times* bestsellers *The Bulletproof Diet* and *Head Strong*. We talked about how important hormones are to our sexual health and it turns out quality fats form strong cell membranes and help build sex hormones.

Dave shared, "Quality fats are clean-burning energy sources that keep your body and brain running at maximum capacity. It's time to end the era of fearing fat. Let's look at some of the ways fat actually helps you. Dietary fat contains more energy per gram than any other nutrient, so it's the most effective way to deliver energy to the parts of your body that need it, like your brain. Compared with protein or carbohydrates, fat has the lowest impact on insulin levels. Insulin spikes are what lead to energy crashes and weight gain."

Some of Dave's favorite ways to get healthy fats are *Bulletproof Brain Octane Oil*, avocado oil, coconut oil, dark chocolate, extra-virgin olive oil, ghee, grass-fed beef and marrow, butter from grass-fed cows, krill oil, and pastured egg yolks. I love to get my healthy fats from avocado. On the days I eat a whole avocado I have more energy, think better, and am satiated because fat makes you feel fuller longer. You may be thinking, *Holy cow! A whole avocado?* Yup! What I am not eating are the highly processed grains and sugars which raise insulin levels and make you ravenous.

"Fat slows the absorption of carbohydrates, keeping blood glucose levels under control. When I do eat carbohydrates, I get them from vegetables. Quality fats often contain fat-soluble vitamins A, D, E, and K. Eating fat alongside other nutrient-dense foods will increase the fat-soluble nutrients you absorb from them, too. That's why it's a good idea to eat fat at every meal, and especially with your vegetables," Dave said. If you get your carbs from grains, stick to whole grains, and be sure to have it with some healthy fat.

Lean Protein

Dr. Shemek shared, "Protein is a key player in optimizing our health. Our bodies need it for mood, energy, cognitive function, immune function, cell membrane health and repair, cell and tissue creation and repair, along with the production of hormones and enzymes. Protein balances blood sugar, helps to quell the hunger hormone (ghrelin) and triggers the weight loss hormone (leptin) that tells the brain you've had enough to eat."

Erin Macdonald, RDN, author of, *No Excuses! 50 Healthy Ways to ROCK Lunch & Dinner!* and the creator of the recipes in this book, said, "A complete protein food contains the nine essential amino acids that the body cannot make on its own and must obtain from our diet. Grass-fed beef, pasture-raised chicken, liver, wild salmon, wild shellfish, pasture-raised eggs, Greek yogurt (unsweetened), grass-fed dairy and grass-fed whey protein isolate powder contain all of the essential amino acids. Incomplete proteins do not contain all the necessary amino acids and are found in foods such as: grains, beans, vegetables, fruits, nuts, and seeds. As long as you get a variety of these foods each day, your body will have the building blocks it needs to make protein."

Colorful Carbohydrates

Erin continued:

> Carbohydrates (carbs) have recently replaced fat as the nutrition devil. With the high-fat/ low-carb movement in full force, you're apt to think that all carbs will make you sick, fat, and definitely not sexy. Let's take a deep breath for a moment and understand what carbs really are and which ones you should be choosing.
>
> Carbs are found in all plants (vegetables, fruits, grains, nuts, seeds, beans) as well as dairy. These are good carbs because they come from real, whole, unprocessed or minimally processed sources. Carbs are also found in sugar, soda, candy, ice cream, cookies, cake, crackers, chips, bagels, waffles, and bread. And the list goes on and on. What you may notice about this list of foods is that they are all sources of processed, refined grains (usually wheat) and high in sugar. Here's the problem. These refined, sugary carbohydrates cause inflammation. They spike your blood sugar level, increase production of insulin, and promote weight gain. Not sexy. And, a steady diet of highly-processed carbs increases your craving for more carbs. It's like being on a roller coaster that keeps going around and around with no end in sight.
>
> The good news is that including the right kinds is carbs at each meal, along with protein and healthy fats, is an amazing recipe for success! Success with your weight. Success with reducing inflammation. Success with lowering your blood pressure, blood sugar, and risk for cardiovascular disease. Success with improving your energy level and reducing your cravings. Success with improved libido, desire, and arousal.

When choosing your carbs at each meal, choose colorful vegetables first. Veggies are full of fiber (which your gut bacteria thrive on) and inflammation-fighting antioxidants and phytochemicals. Erin recommends that you choose at least three different colored vegetables at each meal to ensure a variety of antioxidants. She also suggests that fruit be limited, *not avoided*, to a smaller portion because of its sugar content. Berries are our go-to fruit.

Erin continued, "Grains are a tricky subject for many people. Whole grains such as brown rice, oats, whole wheat, and corn are difficult for many people to digest and may actually contribute to inflammation. Pseudograins, such as quinoa, amaranth, and buckwheat, and sprouted grains may be better tolerated."

Erin will often recommend to her clients that they go grain-free for two to three weeks and see if they notice an improvement in their symptoms, weight, and energy levels. If they do, then they can slowly introduce grains back into their meals, one at a time, to see which ones they best tolerate.

Erin shared, "When it comes to refined grain foods and foods high in sugar, limit it to a very small portion of the overall diet. I like to follow the 80/20 rule. Eighty percent of your food should come from whole, minimally processed, real foods that have a balance of protein, carbs, and fat. That gives you a twenty percent wiggle room to fit in some really good dark chocolate or whatever floats your boat."

Covering the Bases: Go Alkaline!

Daryl Gioffre, DC, celebrity nutritionist, alkaline diet expert, and author of *Get Off Your Acid* explains the Alkaline Diet:

> Just like your temperature, your blood pH works like a thermostat as it is tightly regulated in a narrow range between 7.35 and 7.45, with the ideal pH resting at 7.4. Your body will do whatever it takes to keep that number steady, because if it deviates by more than one point either way, you cannot survive.
>
> The purpose of eating and drinking alkaline-forming ingredients is not to try to raise the pH of your blood, as many mistakenly believe. Eating alkaline is important because it prevents the body from having to do the regulating on its own.
>
> If you're not getting essential acid-fighting materials in your diet, your body will find another way to get them. Your blood will rob Peter to pay Paul in order to keep blood pH at 7.4. This number is so important, your body would rather rob the calcium from its bones, and magnesium from its muscles, and sodium bicarbonate from your mouth, all in effort to keep your blood pH from veering off course.

80/20 Alkaline Diet

To help your body maintain a blood pH level in the alkaline range, Dr. Gioffre recommends following an 80/20 alkaline diet, "This ratio encourages the consumption of high alkaline foods, but also allows flexibility for those acidic items we find hard to resist. You can still drink your wine and have your cake, and you can eat it, too—so long as it's in your twenty percent."

Alkaline Forming Foods

Alkaline foods should comprise 80% or more of your daily diet and consist of dark green leafy vegetables (chard, kale, microgreens, romaine, spinach, sprouts, watercress), essential fats and oils (avocado oil, black cumin seed oil, coconut oil, extra-virgin olive oil (EVOO), macadamia nut oil, MCT oil, omega-3 fats), cruciferous vegetables (broccoli, cauliflower), sulfur-based vegetables (cabbage, onion, radishes), low-sugar fruits (avocado, coconut, grapefruit, lemons, limes, pomegranate, tomato), green juices, green smoothies, green soups, plant-based proteins, raw nuts (almonds, Brazil, macadamia, pecans, walnuts) and raw seeds (chia, flax, hemp).

Acid Forming Foods

Acid-forming foods should comprise no more than 20% of your daily diet and consist of animal proteins, artificial sweeteners, dairy, grains, processed foods, sugar, unhealthy fats, and oils (vegetable oils such as corn oil and soybean oil).

Your Pantry Is a Medicine Cabinet

The following lists of foods and spices not only promote sexual health, they proved additional benefits and are grouped by those specific health goals. Some appear in more than one category.

Natural Antidepressants

Nature's antidepressants include apples, avocados, bone broth, cayenne, dark chocolate, maca, onions, strawberries, and tuna.

Hormone Balancing

Hormone balancing foods include almonds, bone broth, kimchi, kombucha, sauerkraut, tuna, and yogurt.

Increased Stamina

Foods that will boost stamina include apples, bananas, bone broth, shrimp, tuna, and water.

Sexual Health

Foods to enhance sexual health include almonds, apples, artichokes, asparagus, avocado, bananas, beets, black raspberries, blueberries, bone broth, carrots, cayenne, celery, chia seeds, chili peppers, cinnamon, dark chocolate, dates, figs, garlic (raw), ginger, grass-fed beef, kale, kimchi, kombucha, maca, nuts, oats, olives, onions, oysters, pomegranate, pumpkin seeds, quinoa, saffron, sauerkraut, sesame seeds, shrimp, spinach, strawberries, sweet potatoes, tea, tuna, water, watermelon, wild salmon, and yogurt.

Part Three

THE BEDROOM BLUES

I went through high school clueless about sex. I was a late bloomer physically, my mother and I never had "the talk," and in high school my friends kept their sex lives from me to protect my innocence.

The first social humiliation I felt about my sexual ignorance happened at a birthday party sleepover when I was eleven. "Saturday Night Fever" was all the rage—of course I hadn't seen it. While I sank into my sleeping bag, pretending to be asleep, all of the girls at the party were talking about that "Total fox!" John Travolta. Then one of the girls said, "Remember the part when that girl put a bunch of rubbers in John Travolta's hand? I bet Lisa doesn't even know what rubbers are!" Everyone laughed. They were right—I had no idea what rubbers were. I stayed quiet and felt the sting. It hurt. This was not even the low point of the party.

The most humiliating moment of my life happened earlier that evening, setting the stage for my self-esteem and sex issues. The all-girl sleepover started out as a boy/girl party. It was the first time I had been invited to a boy/girl party and I remember getting ready for the evening like it was yesterday. Looking at myself in the mirror, I felt uncharacteristically confident with my newly cut feathered hair and brown and orange patterned shirt (remember, it was the '70s).

Once all the girls and boys arrived, we went downstairs to the basement. At first, the boys were on one side of the room and the girls on the other. After some time, someone shouted out, "Let's play Truth or Dare." We sat in a circle and the game began. Boys were daring each other to kiss certain girls and everything was going fine—until it was Danny's turn. Danny said, "Ron, I dare you to kiss Lisa." Everyone laughed. It was a joke—I was a joke. An unkissable, ugly joke. It was such an outrageous dare that they laughed it off. Not a single girl stood up for me. They laughed too (had my best friend Cindy been there, she would have been in my corner.).

Ron got the "real" dare, and the game continued. The other dared kisses of the evening went smoothly. I wanted to run out of the room. I wanted to disappear. But I sat there, not saying a word. Unkissable me.

That night confirmed something I had been feeling since first grade—I was a loser. There was no place I found solace. At home, in the midst of daily fighting, my sister and I were my mother's caretakers, and at school, both in and out of the classroom, I was a loser.

It would be three long years before I finally started dating at fourteen.

Thinking we'd hit it off, my friend Debbie introduced me to her gorgeous sixteen-year-old ex-boyfriend Steve. So there we were in her backyard, and I managed to pull a cat impression and get stuck in the tree—props on the cautioning Mom. With no firefighters in sight, Steve volunteered. As he helped me down he planted one on me. Holy Moly! I was shocked. We started dating.

For two months our dates consisted of parking and kissing. Finally, he invited me over to his house for our first date at night! I told my mother we were going to the mall. We were sitting on his bed and I was about to make my move when he said, "Let's go to a party." I'd asked Steve if he had a friend for my best friend Colleen, and he said Phil would be a good bet and we should talk to him—once at the party, he told me Phil was in the den. The lights went off the moment I entered the room. Startled, I went towards the door but Phil grabbed me before I had the chance to bring up Colleen, and had his tongue in my mouth. I pushed him away and said, "What are you doing? I'm with Steve!" He said, "Steve thought you and I should go out." What was going on! I stormed out of the room and found Steve, who was sitting with a very pretty girl who told me that she and Steve wanted to get back together and I should go out with Phil. What is wrong with these people?! For me, the party was over. Steve dropped me off and that was that. I was crushed. I wished we had just gone to the mall.

My luck changed at fifteen. I met a guy at a friend's party. He was nineteen going on twenty; I had just turned fifteen, going on twelve. When he approached me and started talking, I was shocked. He was gorgeous, smart, and funny. He asked for my number and shortly thereafter we started dating. It was obvious that I was clueless about sex and all we did was French kiss.

A few months into dating, I invited him over; my parents were away for the weekend and my siblings were out for the night. I still remember what I was wearing—a camisole and jeans. We went to my room, got on my bed and began kissing. About ten minutes in he said, "I need to go." I tried to get him to stay but he politely refused, and left. The next day he broke up with me. I was crushed and felt even less desirable than usual. We really liked each other and his sudden exit reinforced my fears—I was a loser. I discovered years later via Facebook that he left because he knew I wasn't ready for a sexual relationship—I was gratified that he remembered the camisole!

Things began to change for me the summer after high school. I finally went through puberty. No joke! I had a rockin' bod and some self-confidence after the yoga and swimming. For the first time in my life I had numerous dates that summer, but still no action.

On my eighteenth birthday, I received oral sex for the first time—best birthday present ever! I met him while on a camping trip with my family. I wanted to have sex with him and I told a girl I met, who told my older brother, who talked me out of it. To make sure my decision stuck, my older sister drove me outta there under the cover of darkness, station wagon, boat trailer, and red bandana trailing behind. I wish I had done it with him—he knew how to get a woman ready!

Finally, just to get it over with, I had sex with a friend in my sophomore year at college. It was not a great first time. I wasn't attracted to the guy and worst of all, there was no foreplay! Right afterwards I called my mother. She had a liberal, nonjudgmental attitude and we had become close during my teenage years. When I told her I finally had sex, she asked, "Did you have a *good time?*" The lilt in her voice made it seem like I told her I went bowling with friends.

Fortunately, I had a few more opportunities to practice with sex, and foreplay, and once I got comfortable having sex, I started to enjoy it. I enjoyed it so much, I began to use it.

I used sex to escape my problems; unfortunately, it became a problem. What I lacked in self-esteem, I made up for with random hookups. The year both my mother and grandfather died and my relationship of six years ended, my sex/love addiction exploded. I attached unrealistic significance to my many hookups. The void I felt when the guy didn't call could only be filled by finding someone else to love me, to approve of me, to validate me.

A chance encounter at a bookstore changed my life. I was immediately attracted, and felt an irresistible pull. I approached. I was hopeful. This seemed possible and gave me peace. It wasn't another guy—it was a book. How novel!

The book showed me how to authentically love myself, how to spot red flags in relationships, and how to end the vicious cycle of using men to fill the void to validate my existence. To do me and be done with me was no longer for me. It was the beginning of a more hopeful future.

While visiting California on vacation from graduate school, mutual friends introduced me to my husband. We knew we wanted to be together after one date. With six months until my graduation, we courted via landline phone calls and email. The day after graduation, I moved back to California and into his studio apartment.

Together, we moved to the East Coast and two years later we married. Marriage did not cure my sex/love addiction which morphed into initiating sex to feel better about myself. I was approaching sex as a way to fill me up rather than connect. This dynamic did not work for either of us.

I sought professional help through bioenergetic therapy, a form of psychotherapy that combines talking and body work. This helped me resolve some of my emotions and create a healthier sense of self. As a result of my personal growth work, I now reach out to my husband to share love and intimacy rather than to fill an empty need.

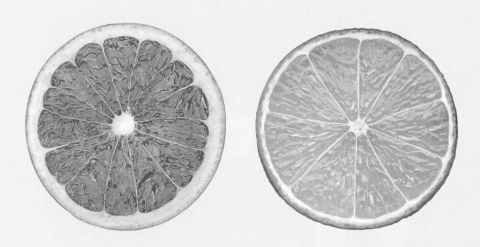

Chapter Five

HORMONES AND SLEEP

We all have estrogen, testosterone, and progesterone in different ratios. Estrogen and progesterone dominate the female sex hormone landscape. Testosterone is important in women for muscle and bone strength, circulation, and maintaining a healthy sex drive.

Testosterone is the dominant male hormone. Younger men generally have higher levels of testosterone and lower levels of estrogen. With aging, estrogen levels often increase and testosterone levels decrease. This can lead to an increased risk of heart attacks, strokes, prostate enlargement, and prostate cancer in older men. Interestingly, estrogen may play an important role in preventing heart disease in men.

Menopause: Before, During, and After

At forty-three, a switch was flipped and I slammed head first into perimenopause. My life went from BPM (before perimenopause) to APM (after perimenopause) in nothing flat. Previously a sound sleeper, I started waking up covered in sweat. I morphed into an angry monster causing my family to flee. Belly weight—that was new. Plus my overdrive sex drive had its license suspended indefinitely.

I longed for balanced hormones. I decided to take action. I saw a doctor who specializes in hormone replacement and had my hormone levels tested. I was low in estrogen and progesterone and I thankfully started hormone replacement therapy.

I asked Hormone Health Educator Candace Burch, MA, to share her vast knowledge about all things hormone. She recommended we start by looking at an overview of hormones during the course of an average woman's life.

Premenopause: The PMS Years

During their twenties and thirties, women should experience fairly regular cycles with balanced estrogen and progesterone production. But increasingly, younger females prone to excessive exercising, stress, crash dieting, and contraceptive use are not ovulating regularly. Anovulatory cycles (menstrual cycles, in part characterized by the absence of ovulation) are associated symptoms of hormonal imbalance, severe PMS, and infertility. They are also common in women with polycystic ovarian syndrome (PCOS).

Perimenopause: The Rollercoaster Years

In the years approaching menopause, forty-something women begin to experience erratic cycles, as ovaries start to sputter, estrogen and progesterone levels fluctuate dozens of times a day. A whole new world of symptoms, from hot flashes and mood swings to insomnia and low libido, take women on a hormonal rollercoaster ride.

Perimenopausal Symptoms

Here is a partial list of symptoms of perimenopause from Candace's website.

acne breakouts/cystic acne

bleeding changes

decreased libido

fatigue

foggy thinking

headaches

hot flashes

incontinence

irritability

memory lapses

mood swings

nervousness

night sweats

sleep disturbances

sugar cravings

tender breasts

vaginal dryness

weight gain

Dear Libido, Why Did You Leave Me?

The consistent major complaint I hear from perimenopausal women is lack of libido. Candace shared one of her posts from her blog *Dear Libido, Why Did You Leave Me?*

> *Dear Libido,*
> *Why did you leave me? And what do I have to do to get you back in my life?*
> *—No Mojo*

Dear No Mojo,

You just might be walking around with an undetected hormone imbalance that's been sabotaging your sex life. *Why*, and how does this happen? Well, hormones work in synchrony to maintain balance sort of like an orchestra, where if one instrument is out of tune the whole symphony suffers. Or like a seesaw, where too much weight at one end causes the board to swing wildly back and forth before it eventually slams to the ground.

And so it goes with hormones—take testosterone, the hormone we all associate with the drive, desire, and libido of the species. Potent though it is meant to be, testosterone has to take a back seat to cortisol, the master stress hormone that when operating in overdrive will make us too tense or tired for lovemaking. When stress hormones stay stuck on the high end of normal for too long, it is not unusual for the hallmark symptoms of hormone imbalance to set in: mood swings, insomnia, headaches, and feeling generally annoyed, impatient and definitely *not* in the mood.

Another all too common libido-lowering scenario is estrogen dominance, a situation where estrogen levels are too high relative to too low levels of progesterone, its balancing partner. This classic imbalance tends to trigger overproduction of a protein known as SHBG, or Sex Hormone Binding Globulin—you don't have to remember that! But what you do need to understand is that when there are too many SHBG proteins around on account of excess estrogens, they actually deplete testosterone making it unavailable for the heavy libido lifting. At the same time estrogen dominance also runs interference on thyroid function, blocking or slowing it down leading to lethargy, weight gain, depression, and other low-thyroid culprits, none of which do much for one's libido.

So my considered advice is to find out if you have a hidden imbalance that may be dimming your desire by testing your hormone levels as soon as you can say 'saliva test.' This is the most convenient, stress-free, and painless (no needles) way to measure hormone levels. Saliva and blood spot tests too can measure bioavailable or 'free' hormone levels to help identify which hormones are actively at work in your body, and which are playing hooky. Shedding a light on this hormonal playing field can illuminate long ignored imbalances that may not only be the culprit behind a libido gone AWOL but a number of other unwanted symptoms you had no idea were caused by a hormone imbalance.

Getting tested is the way to go. When I got tested both my estrogen and progesterone were low. I got on the right hormone levels and I became my sunny self again.

Menopause: The End of Periods

As the ovaries take their final bow, ovulation ends and menopause begins. Falling levels of estrogen, progesterone, and testosterone trigger unexpected symptoms that can surprise women. With less hormone to go around, their role in protecting the health of the uterus, breasts, bones, skin, brain, and heart is greatly diminished. Now is the time when learning to balance hormones becomes more important than ever.

Stress and Sex Hormones

According to Candace, "When stress is prolonged, adrenal hormones start fluctuating up and down, triggering blood sugar and insulin imbalances, food cravings, weight gain, and sleep disturbances. Adrenals under pressure create imbalances of other hormones, e.g., stealing progesterone away from its reproductive duties to make extra cortisol, or inhibiting thyroid function and metabolism.

"If stress levels stay high, the adrenals remain in 'survival mode' to keep us going: by increasing alertness (i.e., sleeplessness), appetite (i.e., overeating) and fat reserves (i.e., stored as belly fat), while sex drive, health, and immunity against illness and disease steadily weaken."

Diet and Sex Hormones

Dr. Masley said, "Guys on an ultra-low-fat diet can create sexual dysfunction by dropping testosterone levels fifty to seventy-five percentage points. In other words, you need healthy fats to have great testosterone levels."

A lack of adequate/complete proteins and healthy fats in the diet can also disrupt female hormones. According to Candace, a SAD diet "raises blood sugar levels which in turn raise insulin levels. High insulin can trigger the ovaries to *over*produce DHEA and testosterone, leading to excess androgen levels that run interference on estrogen and progesterone production. This is strongly associated with formation of cysts on the ovaries, i.e., PCOS."

Get Your Zzz's: Hormones and Sleep

Did you hear about the new corduroy pillow cases? They are making headlines all over town! All joking aside, I take sleep very seriously. When 8:30 p.m. rolls around, I'm in bed with a white noise machine on, earplugs in, and the black-out curtains tightly drawn. I recommend that you get to bed no later than 10:00 p.m. (9:00 p.m. if you hope to *get lucky*).

America's Sleep Doctor™ Michael Breus, MD, wrote in his blog *Testosterone, Sleep, and Sexual Health*, "Changes in testosterone levels occur naturally during sleep, both in men and women. Testosterone levels rise during sleep and decrease during waking hours. Research has shown that the highest levels of testosterone happen during REM sleep, the deep, restorative sleep that occurs mostly late in the nightly sleep cycle. Sleep disorders, including interrupted sleep and lack of sleep, reduce the amount of REM sleep and will frequently lead to low testosterone levels in both men and women."

Women's hormones can affect sleep patterns, most notably during perimenopause. Low or fluctuating levels of estrogen cause sleep disturbance, hot flashes, and night sweats.

Sleep Apnea

Dr. Breus continued:

> Men with obstructive sleep apnea, an inability to breathe properly during sleep, commonly report low libidos and sexual activity. Men who are struggling with issues related to sexual function should have their sleep evaluated by their physician. The good news is that treatments for obstructive sleep apnea—particularly the CPAP—are safe and effective.
>
> Women are also likely to find their sexual lives negatively affected by obstructive sleep apnea. Several studies have found strong correlations between obstructive sleep apnea and sexual dysfunction in women. As obstructive sleep apnea grows worse, problems with sexual function—including sensation and desire—become more serious.
>
> Women are particularly at risk for undiagnosed sleep problems. Women who are experiencing problems with sexual function should have their sleep evaluated. This works in both directions: women who are being treated for sleep problems—particularly obstructive sleep apnea—should work with their physician to assess the potential effect of their sleep disorder on their sexual health.

Chapter Six

KISS ERECTILE DYSFUNCTION GOODBYE

My friend Chris came by at lunchtime the other day, showing up with a sub sandwich from the grocery store. He also brought a bag of chips, a cola, and a stack of extra napkins. "This is going to get messy," he said with a teasing grin, as he squirted an extra packet of mayonnaise onto his sandwich. He knows that I'm a zealot when it comes to healthy eating, and he loves to push my buttons.

As I warmed up a bowl of veggie-packed chili for myself, I said to him, "All the junk you eat is probably going to shorten your life."

He said, "I'm okay with that." With another big smile, he shoved a handful of chips in his face. I sighed. I decided that it was time to hit him below the belt with something all men fear far more than death. "Hmmm. Maybe you don't care about dying, but did you know that crap you eat could be killing your *sex life*?"

There was a long, long pause. Then Chris did something that surprised me: he took the sandwich out of his mouth, set it down, and said, "Okay, you have my attention." We spent the rest of his visit talking about erectile dysfunction—and I started by sharing Marc's story.

Marc's Story: Destiny Is What You Make It

Marc Ramirez is a crusader when it comes to getting guys to eat a clean and healthy diet. That's because unhealthy eating wrecked his love life, and nearly killed him.

In his teens, Marc earned an athletic scholarship to the University of Michigan (Go Blue!), where he played for the legendary Bo Schembechler. "I was an offensive lineman and considered myself to be a man's man," he told me. "I was big and strong, and at 6'2" and 305 pounds, I thought I was invincible."

Marc's Wake-Up Call

Then, as a young adult, Marc began to realize how fragile health and life can be. "My family, which totaled eight brothers and sisters, struggled with chronic illness—mainly type 2 diabetes. We've battled heart disease, cancer, blindness, amputations, organ transplants, dialysis, and years of being unhealthy."

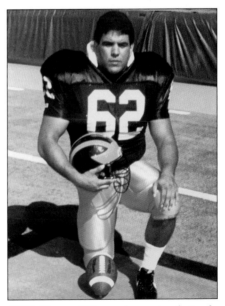

1989. Marc at 305 pounds, a senior playing for the University of Michigan.

The same year his mother and oldest brother passed away, Marc was diagnosed with type 2 diabetes. He wasn't surprised. "After all," he told me, "everyone in my family, with the exception of one sister, has type 2 diabetes. This was in my genes and there was not much I could do about it, or so I thought."

Fast forward another ten years to 2011. "In addition to diabetes," Marc said, "I also had high blood pressure, high cholesterol, psoriasis, frequent heartburn, and weight problems. I was taking five medications every day."

To add his troubles, Marc developed erectile dysfunction (ED). "I would look for any reason to justify my inability to perform sexually," he said, "I even went so far as to blame our dog, and made him leave the room—Sorry, Max!"

He added, "It was very frustrating as a man knowing I could not make love to my wife. It was taking a toll, and I was wondering what was wrong with me. Here I had a beautiful, sexy wife and yet I could not hold up my end of our intimacy."

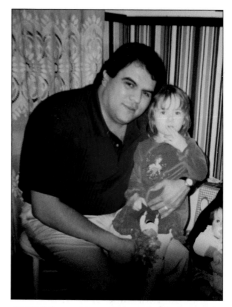

1997. Marc at 280 pounds—already overweight, diabetic, and beginning to suffer from ED.

Marc Answers His Wake-Up Call

On December 3rd, 2011, Marc adopted a whole food, plant-based, clean-food diet. That day he said goodbye to his fast-food diet and his sex life took a big turn for the better.

"I began to lose weight immediately and see my glucose levels drop," he told me. "Within two months I was off all my medications I had taken for the last ten years, even my insulin shots. I also lost fifty pounds in three months. It was very liberating to see how quickly my body began to heal itself."

A few months after changing his lifestyle, Marc got another big surprise, "I was so relieved to see my sexual performance return. I now feel like I am back in my twenties. I once again feel like a man's man."

Today at fifty years old, still medication-free and in the best shape of his life, Marc gives lectures in which he talks openly about ED and other diet-related issues that affect men. He told me, "I do this in an effort to let people know that if you're having

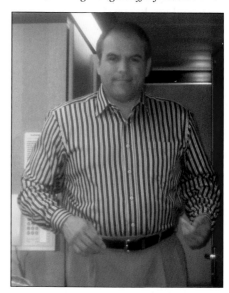

2011. 260 pounds—diabetic for ten years, coping with high blood pressure, high cholesterol, ED, psoriasis, frequent heartburn, obesity, not sleeping well, and taking five medications including insulin shots.

ED issues, you need to address the underlying cause and not just put a Band-Aid on it. If you think you're going to take a pill and all is okay, you might be surprised one day by a heart attack or stroke."

He added, "I'm surprised by how many close acquaintances approach me after a talk and tell me that they're having issues in this department." His message to these men is simple, "You just need to fuel your body with the right foods to keep it up. This is my new mantra: Eating plant based has kept me hard below the waist."

Erectile Dysfunction at Large

Marc's courage in talking openly about his ED is rare, but his story isn't. According to the Massachusetts Male Aging Study, 52% of men over the age of forty experience ED at times. Of these men, 5% to 15% suffer from near-total impotence.

After an episode of ED, men tend to lose self-confidence. Suddenly, that tumble in the hay they used to love becomes a grueling test that they're terrified of flunking. Men with ED often develop symptoms of anxiety or depression, and may start to avoid their partners both in and out of the bedroom. This can cause a serious rift, especially if the partner doesn't realize that the problem is ED.

ED and Heart Disease

Erectile dysfunction involves far more than poor performance in bed. In fact, you should think of ED not just as a sex-spoiler but also as a screaming siren alerting you to mortal danger. In the words of cardiovascular expert Joel Kahn, MD, author of *The Whole Heart Solution*, "ED is the first clue that America's number-one killer is at your doorstep."

According to Dr. Kahn, ED starts with sick arteries. He explains that there are 50,000 miles of arteries in the body, supplying everything from the heart and the brain to the sex organs. These arteries have a single-cell-thick "wallpaper" called the *endothelium*.

When a man's delicate wallpaper gets damaged, Dr. Kahn said, it leads to *endothelial dysfunction*—the cause of 80% of cases of erectile dysfunction. As

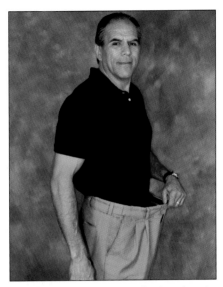

2012. Marc three months after he adopted a whole food, plant-based lifestyle—he was off all medications in two months, and lost fifty pounds in three. He immediately felt slim, healthy, and like a "man's man."

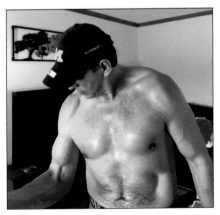

2018. Marc at 208 pounds and in the best shape of his life. He has been medication-free for more than six years and the weight has not returned—he said, "I eat a bunch of food, but a lot of real food."

Dr. Kahn put it, "ED equals ED." Worse yet, endothelial dysfunction puts a man at serious risk for a heart attack or stroke.

Normally, endothelial cells release an enzyme needed to produce *nitric* oxide, a magic molecule that's a real-life love potion. Nitric oxide causes the smooth muscle in the arteries of a man's penis to relax, increasing blood flow and causing an erection to occur.

Unfortunately, a sick endothelium can't produce enough nitric oxide. As a result, the arteries in the penis can't relax and expand. It makes an erection harder to come by, and harder for him to keep it up long enough to do the job.

In the same way, endothelial damage in other arteries, for instance, the ones that supply the heart, prevents these vessels from relaxing in a healthy way. The arteries that supply the heart are bigger than the arteries in the penis, so it takes longer for them to start sending out an SOS when they're hurting. Often, there's no sign of trouble at all until a guy winds up in the emergency room . . . or dead. That's why I say ED is not just sexually debilitating, it's the "canary in the coal mine" when it comes to heart disease.

This is very scary stuff, and it tells you why a prescription for Viagra® or Cialis® isn't the answer. A pill might temporarily seem to fix the problem, but even if his impotence is gone, his blood vessels will keep getting sicker and sicker and that deadly heart attack or stroke will keep inching closer and closer.

So a pill isn't the solution and neither, of course, is giving up on sex! Instead, a man needs to *fix* his blood vessel damage. He needs to heal his endothelium, so his body can crank out that sexy nitric oxide like crazy. And he needs to make those blood vessels that feed his heart happy and healthy, so he can live a long life.

Luckily, as Marc Ramirez's story shows, your guy can do this. He can get back his mojo *and* save his heart. And he can do it all with food and lifestyle changes.

Dudley Danoff, MD, a leading UCLA urologist, recently told me that he sometimes prescribes Viagra® and Cialis® as a temporary bridge while men cure their ED naturally. He said, "It's amazing how many come to me later, and when I ask if they need a renewal of their prescription, they say *no*. These men are getting erections under their own power, they feel great about themselves again, and they don't need that pill anymore."

Science Says

The American Journal of Clinical Nutrition, in the January 2016 edition, published a study involving more than 25,000 men since 1986. Researchers collected dietary data every four years and asked the guys if they could have and maintain an erection strong enough for intercourse. The study found that a higher intake of fruit—especially strawberries, blueberries, red wine, apples, pears, and citrus—was associated with a 14% reduction in the risk of ED (that's why Dr. Kahn calls strawberries "screwberries" and blueberries "blowberries!").

Chapter Seven

MIA—MISSING INTIMATE ACTION

In her TEDx talk titled "The Sex-Starved Marriage," popular relationship therapist Michele Weiner-Davis shared, "When scientists look at the functional MRIs of people who've had a recent divorce or are broken-hearted because of a break-up, the exact same regions of their brains light up as in people who are experiencing physical pain. The same is not true for other emotions like sadness, anxiety, and fear . . . As human beings, we are hardwired for connection. Our need to connect to people we love is more basic and more fundamental than our need for food and shelter."

Plugged into the Distraction Universe

"The fundamental part of sexuality is human connection. It's not about the selfie. It's not about the social media aspects of a relationship. It's really about human interaction, the most important aspect of which is communication," said urologist Deepak Kapoor, MD, president of the Advanced Urology Centers of New York, one of the largest urology practices in the US.

Dr. Kapoor shared, "When I'm with my partner, I'm with my partner. I don't announce, 'I'm putting my phone away,' I just do it. Our time together is our time together. We build intimacy and have shared communication. Intimacy is something you work at and build—it's not something that just happens. It's like the physical aspect of smiling. If you smile and you continue to smile, it causes a biochemical change in your brain and after a while you actually are happier."

Chronic Daily Stress

According to Jennifer Wider, MD, women's health expert, author, and radio host,

"Chronic stress can wreak havoc on your sex life in several ways. When we are stressed, our bodies produce a hormone called cortisol. At high, sustained levels, studies have shown that cortisol interferes with a healthy sex life by lowering our body's libido and sexual arousal. In some people stress interferes with the body's ability to climax.

"In addition, chronic stress has been linked to menstrual irregularities in women, which can negatively impact the libido. People who are chronically stressed have higher rates of depression and anxiety, both conditions are linked with a less satisfying sex life. For people who turn to alcohol to cope with stress, the effects of alcohol can further impair your sex life by causing dehydration which can lead to lower vaginal lubrication and pain during sex."

Balance Your Mental Blocks

"What's in your head goes to your bed," shared Dr. Keesha Ewers, an integrative medicine expert, doctor of sexology, and best-selling author. Our attitudes and beliefs about sex, gender, and sexuality influence our sexual self-expression and experience. Exploring your beliefs and attitudes can yield valuable insights. Once you identify outdated beliefs and self-defeating attitudes, you have the power to change them.

Kim Anami, sex and relationship coach, shared:

It's important to clear anything that blocks women from fully tapping into their sexuality . . . Common blocks for women in our modern culture are . . . that women aren't really allowed to be sexual. There's much more permission given to men to openly own their sexuality and wear it. But for women, there isn't. One of the things to be looking at is the potential ways that you have taken on cultural oppression and internalized it, and it has become a block that one needs to work through.

I encourage people to really look at their sexual energy as a vital, necessary component of their lives and of their relationships. Sexual energy creates life force energy and if you're not creating babies with it you can use it and channel it into your day-to-day life, and use it in your creative projects, and in your work, and parenting, and your relationships at large—and your entire existence.

I get people to reframe their ideas about what sex is, because we live in a time globally where sex has so much baggage attached to it. I believe that we're all innately, naturally sexual beings and that's a healthy, vital, even spiritual part of our existence. So I really have to try to persuade people to understand that this great sexual energy is a great power source for them, especially for women. It's important we accept this sexual side of ourselves and embrace it with openness and honesty.

Resentment and Emptiness

Steven Stosny, PhD, founder of Compassion*Power*, author, and media consultant on relationships, anger, and abuse, shared his thoughts on the major factors that inhibit healthy intimacy:

When resentment is high in committed relationships, sex life almost always suffers. To have a good sex life you have to be able to let down defenses and resentment doesn't let you do that. Regardless of what caused it, you've got to replace your resentment with your core value—your ability to create value and meaning in your life, which is more important than everything you resent.

Core value is the immune system of the self, protecting you from environmental pathogens. When your core value is high you see other people's behavior as a reflection of how they feel. When your core value is low, you're likely to interpret everything as a deep insult. When your core value is low, you're going to be more demanding of your partner because you'll feel like your partner has to pour value into you. It feels like you have a big hole that your partner has to fill. If you perceive yourself to have big holes that someone else has to fill, you're likely to find someone with small cups to fill those holes. That's because people with big cups—a lot of love to give—aren't looking for big holes, they're looking for other big cups so they can get as much as they give. People with small cups—not much love to give—look for big holes who will settle for what little they have to give.

Core value fills your holes and lets compassion, kindness, and love pour out of you. Instead of needing a big cup from someone else, you become a big cup and are more likely to attract others who are compassionate, kind, and loving.

Under the Influence of Unhealed Trauma

When Dr. Keesha asked, "Is there a traumatic experience from childhood that you believe is being activated in your current day relationship and that's affecting your level of libido?" eighty-eight percent of the women surveyed responded "Yes".

Through her 2013 Healing Unresolved Trauma (HURT) survey, Dr. Keesha discovered that the areas of the brain that are impacted by trauma are the same areas of the brain needed for sexual desire and response.

Hypervigilance is one result of child abuse and a symptom of post-traumatic stress disorder (PTSD). Dr. Keesha said, "A hypervigilant mind equals a hypervigilant immune system. This stress response impacts your hormones: perceived threats and fearful thinking means your hormones are in an uproar. This has everything to do with women's libido levels, women's vitality and hormone levels. The sympathetic nervous system activates when there's a threat, so you go in to fight-or-flight mode. Some of the hormones necessary for sexual desire are co-opted by this fight-or-flight system. Your body knows that when it's threatened, it's not safe to have sex."

Dr. Keesha experienced a period of no libido during her marriage—it was twenty years ago and at the time she was newly diagnosed with rheumatoid arthritis, an autoimmune disease. As she drilled down to the root cause, she uncovered repressed memories of being sexually abused as a ten-year-old girl. She shared, "I was wired with a ten-year-old girl's pain. I needed to rewire my sympathetic nervous system's response, tune down that hypervigilance, let my cells know that the messaging they received when I was ten years old was outdated. I needed to upgrade my operating system. So I did. I worked really hard at this. This is not magic pill stuff, it is hard work."

Once she figured out how to heal from the abuse, her autoimmune disease symptoms disappeared. Dr. Keesha developed a program to help others free themselves from the debilitating effects of autoimmune disease and trauma.

When Comfort Is Food

Julie M. Simon, psychotherapist, life coach, author, and creator of the seven-skill mindfulness practice called Inner Nurturing, spoke with me about the crucial role that our early social and emotional environment plays in the development of imbalanced eating patterns.

Julie said, "When we do not receive consistent and sufficient nurturance in infancy and early childhood, our brain and nervous system can become *wired* for high reactivity. This makes it more difficult for us to soothe ourselves and leaves us at greater risk of seeking comfort from external sources, such as food, alcohol, and sex, later in life. Despite logical arguments, we have difficulty modifying our behavior because we are under the influence of an emotionally dominant part of the brain."

Julie shared, "It's our inner world of emotions, bodily sensations, needs, and thoughts that drive our behavior, yet most of us have never had any instruction or education in exploring this inner world. Navigating our often-turbulent inner landscape doesn't come naturally to us. Just as we need music lessons to hone our musical talents and coaching to improve our athletic abilities, we actually need to have certain experiences in childhood or later that help us develop this important skill."

Julie teaches others to *establish the habit of self-connection* by learning to mindfully identify their emotions, bodily sensations, needs, and thoughts. She also teaches how to develop and strengthen an inner supportive voice ("inner nurturer") capable of reassuring and comforting the youngest part of us ("feeling self") and helping us address our needs.

Julie reminds us that the better-than-good news is that "our history is not our destiny." By practicing mindfulness, our brains can be rewired for optimal emotional health. We can learn to nurture ourselves with the loving-kindness we crave, handle stressors more easily, build resilience, and stop turning to external sources for comfort.

Inner Bonding

Margaret Paul, PhD, is co-creator of the Inner Bonding process and author/co-author of several bestselling books, including her latest book, *Diet for Divine Connection*. Margaret spoke with me about how taking personal responsibility can heal depression, anxiety, and low self-esteem.

Margaret told me, "When we're being neglected or abused we're all alone and we're helpless and there's nothing we can do. This pain is too much for a child to manage alone. What happens during child abuse of all kinds is that most of the time a child learns to dissociate. They leave their body or go up into their head as a coping mechanism. It's actually a very good coping mechanism, but it creates a pattern of dissociating from feelings . . . In order to stay in our heads, and away from painful feelings, we learned to judge ourselves, to turn to various addictions, and make other people responsible for our feelings. These self-abandoning and self-rejecting behaviors perpetuate the disconnection that happened during the abuse."

The "wounded self" is the part of us developed in childhood to cope with unmanageable feelings and the "loving adult" is the part we develop to heal ourselves. Margaret said, "The 'wounded self' is all about having control over getting love and avoiding pain and the 'loving adult' is who we are when we're open to loving ourselves."

The "loving adult" develops as you learn to connect with a source of love, wisdom, and help, and bring that compassion and presence to the feeling part of yourself—what Inner Bonding calls the "inner child." To bring acceptance and compassion to one's feelings can be considered spiritual, psychological, or religious. Since the source of love is self-defined—people of all religious and spiritual affinities, atheists and agnostics, can benefit from the Inner Bonding process.

Inner Bonding teaches you to connect with the feeling part of yourself, the "inner child." Through consistent practice, the "inner child" no longer feels alone. The abused "inner child" heals when we take loving action, replacing self-abandoning addictions and addictive processes of the "wounded self" with compassion and self-responsibility of the "loving adult." Margaret enthusiastically remarked, "As we develop the 'loving adult', we start to develop a place of power within us."

Six Steps to Freedom

Inner Bonding is for anyone with anxiety, depression, or low self-esteem, all of which diminish or prevent intimate loving relationships. Intention is the key to the Inner Bonding process. "With Inner Bonding there are only two intentions. You are either in the intention to learn about love and about truth or in the intention to protect against pain with some sort of controlling behavior," shared Margaret. You need to be in the intention to learn in order to do the six steps of Inner Bonding. By staying open to learning, you experience that you are never alone. This is where fears fall away and you begin to receive all the love and wisdom you need to take loving action for yourself and with others.

Step One is willingness to feel pain and take responsibility for your feelings. In this step, you make a conscious decision that you *want* to take responsibility for your feelings and for learning how *you* are causing your own anxiety, depression, anger, guilt, and shame with your own thoughts and actions.

Step Two is moving into the intent to learn. Invite the compassionate presence of love, your higher self, God, compassion . . . into your heart and choose to be in the intent to learn about loving yourself rather than the intent to protect yourself from pain.

In Step Three, you ask your "inner child" questions, such as, "What am I telling myself that is causing this pain?" and you ask your wounded self questions, such as, "What am I avoiding feeling with my protective, controlling behavior?" As you listen inside for answers, you uncover the false beliefs created in the past and which are causing the current self-abandonment.

In Step Four, you ask your source of love (whatever that is for you), "What is the truth about the thoughts/false beliefs uncovered in Step Three?" and "What is loving for me to do in this situation? What is kind to myself?" You open and allow the answers to come through you in words, pictures, or feelings.

In Step Five, you take the "loving action" based on the information that came through from your guidance in Step Four. Over time, "loving actions" heal the shame, anxiety, and depression that resulted from your self-abandonment.

In Step Six, you evaluate if the loving action was effective. Check in with yourself to see if the pain you experienced at Step One was transformed as a result of taking the loving action. If not, go back through the steps until you discover the truth and actions that bring you peace, joy, and a deep sense of intrinsic worth.

This is not a quick-fix process and it takes an effort to learn and stay with the Inner Bonding process, but it is worth it! By practicing Inner Bonding, you foster self-intimacy which is the basis of intimacy with others. When you begin to live as a "loving adult," you heal your fear of abandonment, rejection, and engulfment.

When we are in a "loving adult" state, we don't have an agenda and we're not attached to an outcome. We are not defining our worth by how we look or by what we achieve. When we learn to define our worth intrinsically, by who we really are, we replace depression, anxiety, and fear with a sense of joy and a fullness of love that you want to express in the world.

Part Four

BEDROCK OF BEDROOM BLISS

When my husband and I first got together we couldn't keep our hands off each other. Then, the demands and stress of work, bills, and a special-needs child had us wondering if we'd ever get our hands back on each other.

My newborn daughter barely slept. Most newborns sleep sixteen to seventeen hours per day. I was lucky if my daughter slept five—and she only slept while on top of me! People told me things would turn around at six weeks—they didn't. She didn't sleep through the night until she was six years old. The less she slept, the less I slept. I became increasingly stressed and depressed, and experienced unhealthy weight loss. My sex drive was non-existent. I was in a downward spiral and had to make a change. I needed to take care of myself so I could care for others.

With the help of a naturopath, some self-care practices, and the support of my husband, I began to feel better. In the early '90s, I found a naturopath who helped me address my food sensitivities. This time out a naturopath helped me combat my stress with diet and supplementation.

My husband, in addition to being his loving and supportive self, helped me take time for myself by locking me out of the house. He encouraged play dates with my friends so they wouldn't forget me—and so I wouldn't forget me. Staying connected to friends and the support they provided was hugely important. It was great to feel like myself.

I continue to lay the bedrock for bedroom bliss by staying physically active, emotionally engaged, turned on, and open to more.

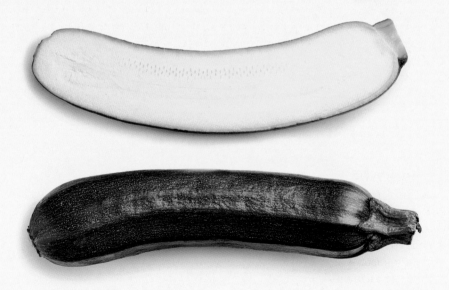

Chapter Eight

MOVEMENT AND CONNECTION

Food and sex are immensely more enjoyable when you are in your body and loving the body you are in. Moving and connecting to yourself is a wonderful prelude to moving and connecting to another. Since cardiovascular health is essential for sexual health, I suggest that you find something you love to do that gets your heart pumping, your body lengthening and strengthening. Do it by yourself, for yourself, or ask your partner to join you!

Dr. Frates reminds us to "Get medical clearance prior to starting any exercise routine."

Let's Get Physical: The Benefits of Exercise

My father played a role in encouraging me to be active in fitness. He ran marathons when I was growing up—lots of training and lots of runs. Sometimes before a long run he would do a shorter route so my sister and I could ride our bikes alongside him. He'd take us back to the house and then continue on. He also played racquetball. I loved that popping sound of the ball when it hit the wall or the floor.

Years later, my dad got into aerobics. I tried aerobics, but being all knees and elbows it was not my cup of tea. I have always enjoyed weightlifting (even without the guys and beefy tostadas) and it turns out I was helping my sexual health.

Boost Testosterone: Lift Weights

Hollis Liebman, author, trainer, fitness magazine editor, and national bodybuilding champion, said, "Although testosterone is widely known as a male hormone, it is also present in females. And like men, as women age, testosterone levels drop, affecting both muscle mass and yes, libido. Studies have shown a correlation between testosterone levels and sexual desire and even performance. Women would do well to add resistance training to their workout regimen to help elevate testosterone levels naturally."

Ted Spiker, professor, chair of journalism at the University of Florida, and former editor at *Men's Health* magazine, shared, "Lifting weights is correlated with boosting testosterone, which is linked to libido. And those are just the physical factors." I reincorporated lifting weights into my fitness regime eight years ago and I have seen an improvement in my physique and my sex drive!

Circulation: What Goes Around Comes Around

Ted stresses the importance of getting your blood flowing by doing cardiovascular exercise. "Exercise improves heart health, arterial health, and overall blood flow, which is one of the main mechanisms for sexual function in men and sexual satisfaction for women."

As discussed above, ED is *a canary in the coal mine*, an early warning system of a circulatory problem in men. With no early warning system, women's first indication of cardiovascular disease can be devastating. This is another important reason for everyone to get up and move.

You can increase your heart rate in so many ways such as biking, running, swimming, dancing, hiking, walking, jumping rope—anything that increases your heart rate. Pick a physical activity that you love so you will be certain to follow through.

Workout Buddy

Ted recommends working out with your partner. "Some couples like to exercise together. Having that shared physical experience works in a number of ways: be it through bonding, or competition, or just being close to each other physically. All of those things can increase hormones that improve various sexual mechanisms. Exercise plays a role in better energy, better moods, better body satisfaction, and all of the things that contribute to how people feel sexually and how people feel engaged in their relationships."

Walking: Baby Steps to Fitness

I was introduced to the joys of dogs as pets, companions, and workout buddies as an adult. I had asked my parents for a dog ever since I was young. I told them it was the only present I wanted for my Bat Mitzvah, but instead they surprised me with a waterbed—harder to walk, but less demanding.

These days my two dogs get me exercising daily. My dogs have a lot of energy to burn, and a fast-paced sixty-minute walk is great for me, and takes the edge off for them.

Even dogless, walking is good exercise. When it comes to making positive fitness and health changes, I believe there is no starting point too low and no step too small. Success builds upon success and before you know it you are off and walking.

Low-impact, almost always convenient, requiring no specialized equipment other than dedicated footwear, walking is a wonderful way to connect with yourself and your partner.

Yoga? Yes, Yoga!

When I was fourteen my mother introduced me to yoga. I was diagnosed with scoliosis and the doctor said it was too late for a brace. The yoga teacher was from India and I loved the unfamiliar aromas wafting through his home. This was my introduction to "exotic" cuisine, aka any food with flavor. My mother was spice-averse; for example, she added only a 1/4 teaspoon of chili powder to a full pot of chili—thank goodness for Rosita's hot sauce. But I digress.

What I didn't love was yoga. It was very hard and it took awhile to get the hang of it. Once I did, I realized that pushing myself out of my comfort zone raised my self-esteem.

I practiced yoga for two years, pleased with my inch-by-inch progression—eventually able to stand on one foot while facing the wall, my other foot high on the wall, with my torso wrapped around my raised thigh.

I didn't set foot on my yoga mat for many years. Pregnancy drew me back when I saw a prenatal yoga DVD by Shiva Rea (that foot on the wall pose seemed like a good delivery position) at the health food store (which smelled wonderful). Daily yoga practice during my pregnancy kept me flexible and strong. I even did yoga on the day of the birth.

As a new mom, I fell off the yoga wagon (is that a pose?). My husband's daily yoga practice inspired me to return to my mat after a fourteen-year hiatus. While my relationship with yoga has waxed and waned, my love of curry and all manner of spice has remained constant.

Yoga Revealed

Despite the images portrayed in the media, you do not need to be impossibly slender, achieve "yoga arms," or sit on a yoga mat, twisted like a pretzel overlooking a tropical blue ocean to enjoy the benefits of yoga.

Yoga is a series of poses, done with focused breathing designed to strengthen and lengthen all the muscles in the body. Moving through poses with the breath is designed to eliminate stress and cultivate self-awareness and presence, or as I like to think of it, feeling calm and staying centered.

Partner Yoga

Jake Panasevich teaches "Yoga for Dudes" and said yoga revitalizes and opens the body which can translate into improving your sexual relationship with your partner. He is an advocate of couple's yoga and recommends couples practice specific partner yoga poses.

Jake and I spoke about the non-verbal communication of partner yoga that can take your connection to a higher level. Wearing comfortable clothes, making physical contact while feeling each other breathing—that's a lot of intimacy. I recommend the seated wide leg twist as a gentle beginner partner pose.

"Shall We Dance?"

When I was in high school my mother and father would dress up weekly—she in one of her crinoline-lined skirts and he in a matching shirt—load up the ice packs, grab my mom's "butt seat" (a portable back support), and off they'd go to square dance.

My sister is a longtime member of the same-sex partner dance community, so I've known of the tremendous health benefits for years. Dance promotes weight loss and improves balance, coordination, core strength, cognitive memory, and circulation. It lowers blood pressure, and reduces stress and stress hormones. Robin Miller, MD, coauthor of *Healed: Health & Wellness for the 21st Century* and *The Smart Woman's Guide to Midlife and Beyond* adds that partner dancing improves cognitive function which results in a dramatic decrease in the risk of dementia and enhances neuroplasticity in the brain.

The psychological benefits of partner dancing include the opportunity to increase social interaction, confidence, self-awareness, and mindfulness. Debbie Ramsey and Wesley Boz, co-owners of Music and Dance Productions, one of the top master West Coast swing instructors in the US, told me, "Dance is another way to communicate without using words. In many ways, it's like sex. There are things that happen with the physical contact and the eye contact, and without even knowing, you're giving in to that deeper communication."

Debbie enjoys dancing with multiple partners. "It's fun, and at a class or dance it allows you to flirt and feel attractive without being unfaithful to your partner. She called it a 'three-minute relationship.' Wesley simply said regarding the romance aspects of dancing, "We advertise, 'If you want romance, learn to dance.' I met my wife dancing. Enough said."

Chapter Nine

CLOSE ENCOUNTERS: ADVENTURES IN INTIMACY

Allow me to introduce three intimacy essentials that, when used with regularity, will deepen your connection and increase your pleasure. Without further ado, the three T's: Trust, Talk, and Touch.

Trust

Trust is the essential ingredient for intimacy and sex. We want to be able to trust others to be honest and reliable. In order to trust others, we need to be trustworthy with ourselves by trusting "gut" reactions, feelings, and needs.

Begin Within

Dr. Margaret Paul shared some insights into trust in the following passages.

> The foundation of healthy trust is self-trust. How often do you promise yourself you are going to do something and then don't do it? Whether it is be on time, start an exercise program, eat healthier, or cut back on sugar. If you promise yourself you will do something and then you don't do it, you are not being trustworthy with yourself.
>
> This would be like promising a child something and then not doing it. Eventually the child would learn not to trust you. The same applies with your 'inner child.' If you promise yourself that you will take care of yourself in some way and then you don't do it, your 'inner child' learns that there is no 'loving adult' to trust.
>
> We can often feel in our body what is true and what is untrue, yet many of us don't listen to these inner messages. Instead, we put our trust in others and then feel betrayed when others let us down. When we choose to listen to and trust our own inner voice rather than give our power away to others, we will no longer put ourselves in positions to be used and betrayed.
>
> Become aware of the knot in your stomach and trust it. Don't analyze it. Don't tell yourself that it must be your issue. Just accept that something is happening that doesn't feel good to you and then, coming from a loving adult, honor your feeling and decide on the loving action.

Trust to Trust

Dr. Paul continued:

> Trust issues abound in relationships. However, resolving trust issues is not about getting another person to be trustworthy. It's about you becoming a trustworthy person with yourself and learning to trust your inner knowing. Since many of us project onto others

our own inner issues, it is likely that if you are not trustworthy with yourself, you will project untrustworthiness onto others.

Trust is built in a relationship when both people are open to learning rather than controlling through anger, withdrawal, compliance, or resistance. When our intention is to control rather than to learn about what is loving to ourselves and our partner, we can never trust or feel secure with our partner, because if we can control and manipulate him or her, others can too—and that's scary. Only when we believe our partner is with us because he or she wants to be—out of desire and caring, rather than out of fear, obligation, or guilt—will we feel secure and trusting.

The more we trust ourselves, the more open and trusting we can be with our partner. People often hold back from being open with their partners with the implication, 'I can't be open until you prove that I can trust you.' By trust they mean being able to predict their partner's response, guaranteeing that their partners will be loving rather than rejecting.

One of life's hardest realities is that this kind of guarantee is impossible. However, the more we trust ourselves and develop our ability to speak our truth, the more we are willing to be open and risk another's free response to us. This is what creates a loving and trusting relationship.

Pillow Talk

You might recognize the heading from the 1959 movie of the same name. I love those old movies filled with romance and lip-locked kisses. This pillow talk need not require pillows, the bedroom, a telephone, or sex—communication. Verbal communication. You know . . . talking.

Communication is essential for every aspect of a relationship and it's not surprising that the majority of people don't talk about their sexual likes and dislikes. In fact, research shows that the majority of people have no idea what their lover prefers when it comes to the duration of foreplay and intercourse—and the average adult knows only about *one quarter* of his or her lover's dislikes. As a result, couples can go for decades feeling frustrated and dissatisfied.

Talking Points

Here are some strategies for laying the groundwork and initiating an open, honest conversation about sex.

Use "I" messages. "I" messages communicate directly what you want and need and increase receptiveness from your partner. For example, "I would love for us to become more connected sexually," rather than "you" messages like "You don't seem to want sex much anymore." *You* messages are often perceived as attacks, which may elicit defensiveness.

Talk in a private location at a prearranged time. Not in the bedroom, not in the car, and not in emails or texts! Find a time when you and your partner can relax and have time to listen. Open the conversation with a gentle request to talk about intimacy, stay open, and see where the conversation leads.

Be positive and supportive. Approach the conversation as a willing partner. For example, if you know your partner is stressed out at work, say, "I know it's hard to feel romantic when you're working so hard. Is there anything I can do to help?" and, "I know I want sex more often than you; can we talk about a minimum amount per week we can set that is comfortable to us both?"

Be a guide. During sex, speak up! Give your partner both verbal and nonverbal guidance and encouragement! Tell your partner what you like, what you want more of, and what feels good. Guide with your hands, or make some deep exhalations when your partner does something that turns you on. Positive feedback can heat things up. KC and The Sunshine Band got it right with "That's the way, uh-huh, uh-huh, I like it. Uh-huh, uh-huh!"

Do your homework (no cheating). Learn about what you like sensually and sexually in order to please yourself and to communicate your needs and desires to your partner. Get yourself in the mood with dimmed lights, bubble bath, or dance around the living room in a button-down shirt, socks, and underwear. Once you are ready, use your hands, and toys if you like, to explore your body.

Touch Is Essential

Barb DePree, MD, a gynecologist and a women's health provider for almost thirty years, highlighted several behaviors that involve non-sexual touch that release oxytocin and other neurochemicals which "help dispel defensiveness, and make bonding not only possible, but effortless." Some of these behaviors you may remember from when your romance started and include affectionate touch, caregiving, and lots of loving eye contact.

Numerous studies indicate that human touch is essential to our well-being. Most nights of the week, you will find me on the sofa watching TV exchanging gentle back rubs with my husband. It is our way to connect with nonsexual touch. Apparently I am one of the lucky ones.

Patti Britton, PhD, MPH, clinical sexologist, cofounder of Sex Coach University, and author of *The Art of Sex Coaching*, said, "There is a profound lack of physical connection in these relationships. One of the symptoms of a sexually bankrupt relationship is the couple stops touching at all. People aren't being physically touched, so, when they're sexless, they're also touchless."

She asserted we need touch to thrive as humans. Studies demonstrate that people need to have human contact and be touched—it's essential.

Dr. Britton said, "When people are not engaging in sex, they're probably also not hugging. This is because they're afraid that acts of affection might be interpreted as a signal to be sexual when they're not ready for sex. That if they hug, if they hold hands, or if they run their fingers through their partner's hair just before sleep . . . what's going to happen is their partner is going to think it's a signal."

The Touch Continuum: Five Levels of Touch

Dr. Britton shared, "We want sex, but we want to be held, we want to be close, we want to be face to face, we want to feel." Not all hugs lead to kisses and not all kisses lead to sex. Dr. Britton has outlined the touch continuum as five ascending levels:

1. **Healing touch:** very light touch when you are sick, tired, or in pain. Energy work.
2. **Affectionate touch:** expresses friendship, caring, and nurturance. The touch is playful and light.
3. **Sensual touch:** lavishing touch for its own pleasure, or to bring people closer together.
4. **Erotic touch:** intimate touch (akin to "foreplay") such as deep kissing and petting or caressing.
5. **Sexual touch:** can include kissing, but also involves anything two naked bodies can do together.

Dr. Britton teaches couples that they can and should remain at a comfortable lower level until they are both ready to move on. This helps couples experience touch for the sake of connection without sending a message that any touch means go straight to level five. Dr. Britton said, "What's so funny is when they become touchers again, guess what happens? The sex comes back!"

Chapter Ten

TOUCHABLE, KISSABLE SKIN

When I was in my thirties I never gave much thought to age-related skin change; at a cafe, I overheard two women talking about their upcoming Botox party—I rolled my eyes. When I go to a party I like to eat yummy food and chat with friends, and if there's music, I like to dance—not have needles jabbed into my face!

Fast-forward fifteen years and the Botox party is something I'd gladly attend! This chapter is not about Botox, fillers, etc. (I have nothing against them—I use and *love* fillers); it is about being more comfortable in your skin by incorporating these head-to-toe skin care tips.

The idea of beauty from the inside out became important to me when I turned forty and noticed fine lines, wrinkles, and acne. Yup, fun to have all three! The advice I am about to share with you improved my skin dramatically.

I still have crow's feet and the occasional pimple; however, I regularly get complimented on my skin's glow.

Great Skin from Within

Nutritional deficiencies are a very common trigger for skin issues and could indicate a deeper health issue, including inflammation, food toxins, and/or imbalances in gut bacteria. I spoke with Trevor Holly Cates, ND, a naturopathic physician known as "The Spa Dr.," about the connection between diet and skin. Dr. Cates shared, "I see over and over again how the foods people eat impact their skin. You've probably seen it yourself and already know that diet plays a role."

Collagen is an essential protein for health as it literally holds our bodies together. Collagen is in our skin, bones, tendons, ligaments, and joints. Daily collagen intake is essential to promote healthy gut microbiota, and to slow down the aging process. Avocado, berries, bone broth, chia seeds, chlorella (a single-celled algae), eggs, garlic, leafy greens, mango, pumpkin seeds, and wild salmon are all sources of collagen. Remember to eat these with citrus since the vitamin C is needed to knit collagen precursors together.

Bone Broth

Drinking bone broth has been a game changer for my skin. I first heard of all the incredible benefits of bone broth from Kellyann Petrucci, MS, ND, naturopathic physician and weight-loss specialist. Dr. Petrucci shared the top reasons to add bone broth to your diet.

The collagen in bone broth promotes gut health and helps you to maintain proper serotonin levels. Serotonin is a neurotransmitter that helps you feel happy, gives you energy, and makes you feel in the mood to have sex. Studies have shown that 90 percent of serotonin is produced in the gut, demonstrating that gut health and sex hormones are closely linked.

The collagen in bone broth gives you sexier skin. Oral collagen peptide supplementation (drinking bone broth) significantly increased skin hydration after eight weeks of intake.

Glycine is also important for the synthesis of hemoglobin and myoglobin, which transport oxygen throughout the blood and muscle tissue. Oxygenated muscles are crucial to sexual performance. Glycine also improves muscle health by protecting muscles during different wasting conditions, and can also improve sleep quality.

The phosphorus and magnesium in bone broth are essential for muscle performance. Deficiencies in these minerals results in decreased stamina and in some cases increased muscle cramping. A poorly timed muscle cramp can really ruin a lovely time.

Bone broth also restores glutathione, which protects against oxidative stress. It helps keep your hormones in balance by decreasing the impact of bad estrogen buildup.

Bone broth contains the amino acid arginine, which improves blood flow and circulation, which is useful in treating erectile dysfunction. Women benefit from increased circulation and the associated increased sensation as well. Our fabulous bone broth recipe awaits you on page 79.

When Beauty Is Skin Deep

Even though we have been washing our face for most of our lives, there are ways to do these basic tasks that yield better results. Susan Ciminelli, world-renowned holistic health, beauty, and wellness guru, told me, "To avoid damaging the capillaries in your face, wash your skin with a washcloth, use a warm water wash and a cool water rinse."

Susan strongly advised to never use a bar of soap. David Pollock, chemist and beauty industry veteran, agrees. He told me that our skin has an acid mantle, as part of its protective barrier. The skin has a pH of 4.5 to 5.5 which is lower than a bar of soap, which has a pH of 9. A run-of-the-*milled* bar of soap disrupts the skin's natural pH, damaging the skin's natural lipid barrier. This results in dry skin and exacerbates skin problems like rosacea and psoriasis, and even accelerates the signs of aging. Instead of bar soap, use a liquid body and face wash because the pH is closer to your skin's natural pH.

"You Look Marvelous": At-Home Skin Care Routine

Susan offered the following tips for skin care and cleansing that can be done at home.

Cleanse: Choose a lightweight, creamy cleanser that contains hyaluronic acid for extra hydration and keeping pores clean.

Exfoliate: Not only your face, but your entire body. A natural exfoliant like an algae cleanse contains glycogen to remove dead skin cells deep within pores.

Moisturize: Use a moisturizer with shea butter, vitamins A, C, E, and protein. For sun protection, use SPF 30 or higher.

Hydrate: Use a hydrating mask with a skin peel and a nourishing skin-activating serum.

Hollywood Dry Brush Routine: Using a natural bristle body brush, dry brush your body to bring blood to the surface of your skin. Blood carries oxygen which will help burn off the fat layer. Always brush toward your heart. Start at your ankles, do your legs, and move upward. Then take a seaweed bath for up to forty-five minutes.

For makeup, Susan recommended a tinted moisturizer with antioxidants; it'll provide your skin with nourishment to combat free radicals, and prevent wrinkles. For dry skin, cracked elbows or heels, David recommends a heavy moisturizer rich in hyaluronic acid. "Even consider taking a hyaluronic supplement to help hydrate the body from the inside out."

Pampering Professional Facials

In addition to my in-home skin care routine, I started getting monthly facials several years ago because my pores on my nose are so large an extended family of fairies could live in them. The substance that clogs pores and causes acne is sebum. I have a lot of sebum and call myself the sebum queen. Getting the monthly facials has been great for my pores and for my skin.

I adore my master esthetician Michelle Nunez. Michelle said, "Facials aid in blood circulation and lymphatic drainage, reduce puffiness, exfoliate the skin, remove excess sebum which leads to clogged pores and breakouts, and are a great way to relax and unwind. If professional facials are not an option, then I recommend adding a clay-based mud mask to your face care regimen once a week."

Grooming Down Under

Both men and women are getting more creative when it comes to grooming "down under." When it comes to pubic hair, to each their own. After resisting for years, I was hesitant, but finally was fed up with my public hair sticking out of the sides of my underwear. I wasn't up for the Brazilian (where they remove all of the hair) so I tried out the bikini line touch up.

I was so nervous when I showed up at the spa to get waxed. I must have asked the esthetician one hundred times, "Is this going to hurt? How much? On a scale of 1–10? She had another client after me so eventually we had to get on with it.

I'm not going to lie, it really hurt the first few times. The good news is it is less painful over time and when the hair grows in, it's less dense and finer. Now I get waxed once a month. My advice before you remove any pubic hair is read up on the pros and cons of the various methods.

Kick Toxins to the Curb

Before I was educated by my friend and co-host David Pollock, I would buy a lot of skincare products: face wash, moisturizer, serums—you name it, I bought it. Turns out many of them contained harmful chemicals that are toxic and get absorbed through the skin.

When David gave me a list of ingredients to avoid in skin care products, shown below, I took on the task to get the toxic skincare products out of the house. I read every label and poured out anything with toxic ingredients into a bag which I threw in the trash, and rinsed each bottle and put it in the recycling bin. It was a lot of work, but my health is worth it!

David gave me the following list of the top chemicals to *avoid* when buying skin care products. Most of the ingredients are difficult to pronounce and all have detrimental effects on our health.

1. Parabens, also called methylparaben, ethylparaben, propylparaben, benzylparaben, and butylparaben
2. PEGs's & Glycols, also listed as polyethylene glycol (PEG), and propylene glycol

3. Lauryl/Laureth Sulfates, can also be listed as sodium lauryl sulfate, ammonium lauryl sulfate, sodium laureth sulfate, ammonium laureth sulfate (even if it reads "Coconut Derived" or "From Coconut")
4. Petrochemicals, can be called mineral oil, petrolatum, light liquid paraffin, petroleum distillate, mineral jelly, petroleum jelly
5. Synthetic Fragrance
6. Synthetic Dyes
7. Triethanolamine
8. Triclosan
9. Phthalates
10. 1,4-Dioxane

According to the Environmental Working Group (EWG), Americans slather themselves with an average of nine personal care products each day which expose them to one hundred and twenty-six (mostly) toxic ingredients. In Europe, they've banned more than one thousand ingredients in personal care products, but in the United States, only eleven ingredients have been banned by the United States Food and Drug Administration (FDA). It is super important to be aware and educated about the ingredients in our facial and skin care products, because what we put on our skin gets absorbed.

Chapter Eleven
"LET'S GET IT ON"

D^{r. DePree told me, "My birthday is coming up and [my husband and I] made a reservation at a favorite restaurant. I already know what we plan to order. We'll have a great time.}
And I guarantee you, we'll go home and have sex afterward." She went on to explain, "My mom wants to have dinner with me, too, and I thought about inviting her. But then I realized, I can't. It occurred to me that for us, this is foreplay."

Foreplay is an umbrella term for a vast array of activities that are preparation for and anticipation of a sexual encounter, and sometimes it is the sexual encounter!

It's time now to turn up the heat and move toward creating some bedroom bliss. Sex therapist Vanessa Marin, MA, said, "When it comes to sex, especially in long-term relationships, even the smallest changes can make a world of difference."

Time and Privacy: Lovers' Lair

When do you have some private time with your sweetie to be sexually intimate? For me, it's the moment my daughter steps from the curb onto the school bus and before my husband leaves for work; I know I have an hour window to grab my husband and get busy.

Most experts advise you need a safe, distraction-free place to be sexual. This includes freedom from preoccupations with work, housework, kids, projects, deadlines, obligations, and technology. Creating a distraction-free space is yet another reason yoga or another form of meditation and mind-calming is so essential. You need to clear the inner clutter in your mind in order to be present, just as you need to clear off your calendar to make the time for connection.

Mark Kroll, Certified Hypnotist, shared that hypnosis is an excellent tool for helping his clients learn to overcome inner clutter. He explained, "Sometimes the big, important thoughts keeping us from being in the moment *are* big, important thoughts. Other times the inner clutter carries less weight. Regardless the nature of the clutter, it can be difficult to let it go and be present.

My clients learn to pause, breathe, and release cluttering thoughts. One hypnotic technique that facilitates this process is to create a mental locker from which no thoughts can escape. While in trance, the client places all extraneous thoughts into the solid locker, closes the door, spins the dial, and knows right where those thoughts will be should they choose to retrieve them. Once the techniques are practiced, the locker is never more than a deep breath away."

Once you have cleared the inner clutter, in order to have privacy, you need a time when you can be alone with your partner without interruptions (even your phones and other devices). Depending on your living situation, family size, and kids' schedules, this may require getting a lock on the bedroom door, sending kids to a trusted family member's or friend's house, or exchanging childcare with another family.

Priorities: Scheduling Sex

Prior to becoming a TV and radio host, I was a healthy lifestyle coach. In order to prioritize reaching their healthy lifestyle goals, I always recommended my clients schedule exercise, put it in the calendar and do it just like any other appointment. Now I am telling you to schedule sex.

Vanessa Marin, MA, a licensed psychotherapist specializing in all things sex, gave me some great tips, "Scheduling sex helps on a logistical level, but it goes deeper than just blocking off an hour of time in your calendar. It's a way of showing you and your partner that you value your sex life. We schedule the things that are important to us. Why should sex be any different?"

When my husband and I schedule sex, sometimes we just get right to it and other times we make it a date. Vanessa said, "Having a date on the calendar actually creates an incredibly sensual anticipation. You can bring back that element of anticipation. Get gussied up for each other like you used to before your dates. Fantasize about your date throughout the day. Send flirty texts or emails." I agree, flirty texts on a day of a sex date are a big turn on for me!

Stocking the Bedside Table

Once you've set a date, make sure you are physically ready. Not only do you need to bathe, or not, and get dressed, or not, you need to stock your bedside table with everything you want on hand for when you are tangling up the sheets.

Vanessa suggests to stash "nice undies," a bottle of lubricant (my favorite is *Woo for Play*), and sex toys in your bedside table. I always make sure my lubricant doesn't contain endocrine disrupting hormones. When I want an element of surprise, I ask my husband to pick out lingerie for me.

For sex toys, Vanessa recommends a cock ring, like the Je Joue Mio for men and a vibrator for women. Her all-time favorite vibrator is Minna Life Limon. My personal favorite device is the good ol' neck massager aptly named the magic wand!

Vanessa recommends a wedge pillow like the classic Liberator wedge. She also recommends "some basic bondage gear, like a blindfold, a light whip, and a pair of restraints."

Essential Oils

Essential oils not only support a variety of health conditions, from skin conditions and diabetes to digestive issues, they are also a great way to relax and get in the mood.

Heidi Moretti, MS, RD, LN, known as the Diet Detective, shared her love of essential oils: "I rarely go a day without using lavender in some way. Why? It simply is one of the most versatile plants around and practical in so many ways. It's easy to grow, inexpensive to buy, and full of scientifically proven health benefits. Lavender works great for cleansing and it smells delicious. I love it in teas, coffee, and savory dishes. It works in oatmeal and berry spreads. I use it for my laundry and my home humidifier and it is much safer than chemical additives or perfumes. I love the scent. I use it to relax."

My advice: soothe your skin by adding some oil of your choice to a bath along with some drops of lavender essential oil. You will feel soft and relaxed.

Variety Is the Spice of Life

Moving out of one's comfort zone to spice things up requires trust and respect. In my experience, the spice quotient of my married sex life increased as these qualities increased in my relationship.

Vanessa has some hot ways to spice things up: "Most of us default to doing the same activity in bed. For heterosexual couples, it's typically intercourse. Gay and lesbian couples tend to default to intercourse, toy play, oral sex, or manual stimulation."

"Happy Together": Mutual Masturbation

"In my opinion, mutual masturbation is one of the most underrated sexual activities. If you've never tried it before, the name is self-explanatory—you and your partner both masturbate at the same time. You can also take turns watching each other masturbate," Vanessa shared.

Backdoor

This subject is still taboo. Way back when I was single and dating up a storm, only one guy tried to check out mine. Now I read about it, hear about it, and get direct messages on social media from men who say they'd love to play with my butt! It's obviously more popular these days.

Women find their male sexual partners love it once they are willing to try it but there is still a lot of stigma and questions around what it means it terms of sexual preference. Vanessa said, "This should go without saying, but if you identify as straight, exploring anal play doesn't say anything about your sexual orientation. Anal play can feel incredible. You have nerve endings in your rectum and around your anus, so there's just no getting around the fact that it feels good."

You Never Know Until You Try

I have never had a problem initiating sex. Do I always get it? No. Could it be the way I am bringing it up (pun intended)? "Hun, do you want to have sex?" may work some of the time, and Vanessa Marin gives the following tips to increase your positive response rate when initiating sex.

Sweet Memory Lane

Vanessa suggests, "Jot down a list of four or five of your hottest sexual experiences with your partner, then try to look for similarities in how those experiences were initiated. Ask your partner if they have any favorite memories of ways you initiate sex. Share your favorite memories of your partner initiating too." I tried this with my husband and we had a great time strolling down memory lane, and then took a sharp left into the bedroom.

Lavish Compliments

Next, Vanessa continued, "Compliment your partner, your relationship, or the sexual connection the two of you share." This was a natural for me. I love to give compliments! "Make your initiation feel more personal by telling your partner exactly *why* you want them in that moment. Say something like: 'Your ass looks so incredible in those pants. I want to get my hands all over it,' or 'I can't believe how lucky I am to get to look at you every day.'"

Be a Tease

"Drawing out your initiation can be really freaking hot. It gives both of you the chance to prepare for sex mentally and build anticipation. Send your partner a text during the day saying, 'I'm wearing that underwear you love. See you tonight!' Or parade around in said skivvies but tell your partner you're 'off limits' until later that evening."

My friend Bob does something extra special to prepared for a scheduled sex date. The morning of the evening sex date, Bob will pick out a sexy pair of panties for his wife to wear. Wearing them all day builds up the anticipation for them both.

Be Proactive

Because I work in radio I don't dress up, wear make-up, or for that matter, shower most days! Just kidding. I shower. I may be clean but I am always in athletic clothes—day in and day out.

It is all my husband even sees me in. Once in awhile, I like to put on a sexy dress I know he loves or some tight jeans and high black boots. When he comes home and I am looking hot, it helps! I bring this up because Vanessa's next suggestion is to be sexy: "Bust out that move you used to do all the time but haven't in a while. Maybe on your first date, you pushed your partner up against their door and kissed them until you were both panting. Or channel your intensity through your words. Tell your partner, 'I need to have you right now' or 'I've been driving myself crazy thinking about you all day.'"

Have Fun

My husband and I love to joke around. My mother told me to marry someone who makes me laugh. I took her advice. Being playful is a big part of our relationship. Vanessa recommends being playful when initiating sex. "Initiating sex doesn't always have to be so serious! You might feel way more comfortable (and even way more sexy) being silly and playful." Have a code word or phrase for when you are in the mood. Ours is "Supercalifragilisticexpialidocious." Just kidding. It's "Chim chim cher-ee." (Bet you are either singing or humming!)

Chapter Twelve

FEMALE ANATOMY: IN THE HOOD

Vagine, va-jay-jay, honey pot, vag, hoo-ha, yoni—just a few of the names for a vagina. Whether you have brazenly dubbed yours with a *handle* like "Paradise Cove," or meekly refer to it as "down there," the following information can help you maximize your potential for pleasure. The "you" in this section is directed at women. Men, don't skip ahead! If you have a female partner, you'll need this information too!

Clitoris: Tip of the Iceberg

A widely held myth is that the clitoris is a little button. It's not. However, this did not come to light until the 1990s when an Australian urologist, Helen O'Connell, literally looked under the hood and discovered that the clitoris is an enormous wishbone structure filling up the majority of the pelvic region behind the vagina. The button is figuratively the extremely sensitive tip of an extensive iceberg. Under the skin, the clitoris has legs and erectile tissue, and the tip contains eight thousand nerve endings! That's more nerve endings than in a penis. The clitoris has only one function, and one function only—pleasure.

G Marks the Spot

In the female anatomy treasure hunt, G marks the spot. This highly sexually responsive location is known as the Gräfenberg or G-spot. Dr. Britton explains that it is not actually a spot but a region within the vaginal canal.

Dr. Britton suggests that the first time you set out to find it, do so when you are not aroused. This will provide time and space to find it so next time you are aroused, you know where it is.

I found my G-spot when I wasn't looking for it—what an awesome surprise! It was during intercourse when my husband entered my vagina from behind. Since then, it's my sexual position of choice, though I visit the missionary position often for the great kissing!

G-Spot GPS

In order to find the G-spot, a woman, or her partner, dips their finger all the way into the vagina and feel for something that feels like the end of a nose; that's the cervix located at the end of the vaginal canal. You will use the knowledge of the full length of the canal to find the G-spot.

To locate the G-spot area, enter the vagina only about a third of the way from the entrance. Feel into the wall nearest the clitoris, toward the front of the body. The G-spot should feel a little rough, like the surface of a walnut. To make sure you are at the desired location, add some stimulation and if you hit the G-spot, you are likely to get a response.

G-Spot Stimulation

There are many ways and various sexual positions to use in order to provide a woman G-spot stimulation. One technique is for the woman to get on all fours and let the partner enter the vagina from behind. In this position, the G-spot is contacted directly. Another technique is to reach up and move the finger in a come-hither motion. Now that you know the goal, you can research other techniques—or use your ingenuity, or sex toys made for this specific purpose, as you explore.

A New Sexual Response Model for Women

The groundbreaking work of gynecologist William Masters, MD, and sexologist Virginia Johnson, first published in 1966, defined women's sexual response based on a linear model progressing in four stages: arousal, plateau, orgasm, and resolution. In 1979, sex therapist and activist Helen Kaplan, MD, updated and condensed the model to three phases: desire, arousal, and orgasm. Any response by a female outside of that model was pathologized as sexual dysfunction.

The work of Masters & Johnson and Kaplan, has been reviewed over the years by researchers and some of their conclusions have been called into question; although the model fits men, it neither fits women nor considers sexual response in the context of relationship.

Rosemary Basson, MD, from the University of British Columbia, created a new model of female sexual response that is circular, not linear, and includes emotional intimacy, sexual stimuli, and relationship satisfaction.

The Big O–Wow: Variations on a Theme

To better understand the female sexual response, Dr. Basson developed not one, but a series of five models to illustrate the variety and complexity of women's sexual response.

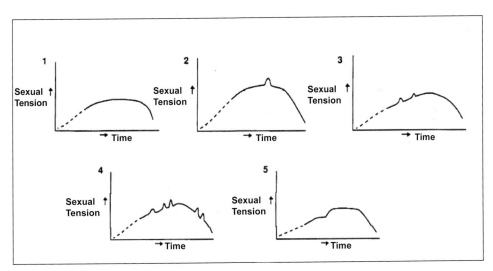

Dr. Rosemary Basson's models for female sexual response.

Some of the models depict multiple orgasms, while others show stimulation with no orgasm. Dr. DePree took these and other diagrams from Dr. Basson's work and interpreted them into a circular diagram and added interpretation of the linear Masters and Johnson and Kaplan model for comparison.

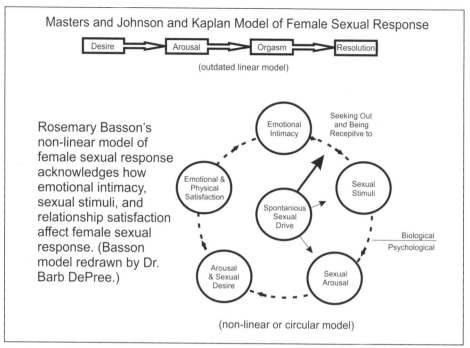

The linear and outdated Masters and Johnson and Kaplan model compared to the Basson circular model for female sexual response.

The two models are very different, and the circular model developed by Dr. Basson sets very different expectations for a woman's response in a sexual situation. Dr. Basson's inclusion of the relational components of female desire and sexual response are key ingredients. As the diagrams show, women's sexual response works non-linearly. Women may go back to previous points in the process, or jump ahead; they are capable of multiple orgasms of varying intensities.

"Sisters Are Doin' It for Themselves"

One of my most embarrassing life moments occurred because I forgot to heed my parents' advice. As a kid, while watching television in the family room, I tended to rock side-to-side on my tummy—it worked like a charm. Unbeknownst to myself at the time, I was masturbating. My parents told me to take it to my room.

I once was in the family room of a friend's house with my friend and her mother. We were watching television. I started rocking, not consciously aware that I was doing it! It was an innocent habit—probably took less than sixty-six days to develop.

My friend's mother, a devout Catholic, was horrified. She told me it was a sin and to never do that again. I was super embarrassed but decided to take my parents' advice instead. I don't think her mother ever looked at me the same way again.

Many of the experts I interviewed agree that self-stimulation, also known as masturbation, is important for women. In order to increase pleasure and comfort with sexuality and sexual expression, a woman needs to know her body. When a woman knows what makes her feel great, she can give herself pleasure and communicate what she likes to her partner. Dr. DePree recommends self-stimulation twice a week, because, like any skill, the more you practice, the better you get.

If you need help getting started, there are actually books on the topic. Breathe, relax, and remember to include foreplay in your solo-play!

Personal Vibrator

A personal vibrator is helpful because the clitoris, if not stimulated, will go dormant, and pull up into the body. Dr. DePree said as you age, you need a vibrator with more *umph*, because it needs to overcome the sluggish circulation in an older clitoris, especially one that hasn't been stimulated in a while. So the vibrator needs to be stronger and able to go longer to replace the circulation the clitoris has not gotten and encourage it to "come out to play."

You may want to try several vibrators for different situations and vibrators that offer other benefits, like ones that also stimulate muscle contraction in the vagina (like Kegel exercises) in order to help intensify your orgasms.

Not Your Granny's Kegels: Vaginal Barbells, Vacuums, and Lasers

Most women have heard about Kegel exercises. The way I was taught to find my vaginal muscles was to stop my urine flow midstream when I went to the bathroom. Once I found them, I was instructed to squeeze them at random times during the day, while waiting at a traffic light, for example. This would stave off urinary incontinence and make sex more pleasurable, or so I was told. I thought I knew all about Kegels, and I was no longer bored at red lights.

Well, I've been enlightened by the experts and I don't want to burst your bubble, but if you are like me, you've been missing an important aspect of the Kegel exercise experience.

In order to get the most benefit from the exercise, you need to use a weight in the vagina to give the muscles something to work against. That is the strengthening part of the exercise, the muscles in the vagina hold the weight so it doesn't fall out. It might sound awkward, but it doesn't have to be.

This weightlifting part of the exercise was intended by Dr. Kegel, who is known for the exercises named after him. Many women who have been religiously doing their Kegels had no idea there was more to it.

Banish Incontinence with Vaginal Kung Fu

On the scale of embarrassment, all the specialists I talked to agreed nothing will hinder a woman's sex life more than the humiliation of urinary incontinence. Pain, burning, and frequent urination (can't hold it or feeling like you always have to go) are the symptoms.

Kim Anami, sex and relationship coach and vaginal weightlifter, likens the kind of Kegel exercises most women are taught to do with going to the gym and standing in front of the weightlifting equipment and flapping your arms and legs, rather than picking up the weights and actually moving them yourself.

Vaginal weightlifting is the modern term for these exercises, and Kim is an expert. When done correctly, with a "weight," it can produce a 90% reduction in urinary incontinence and increases orgasmic pleasure as well. Kim calls it "vaginal kung fu."

Jade Eggs

There are many devices a woman can insert and hold in her vagina to practice real Kegels, or real vaginal weightlifting. Kim said, "The Chinese used a jade egg, a stone carved and polished into the shape of an egg, with a hole drilled through and a string through the hole.

"The way it works is you push the egg into the vagina. Then you hang things from the string. You can start with a 16-ounce bottle of water and increase from there. If it's too heavy, you find something smaller, (or it make lighter by using less water). The idea is to build up gradually. The shower is a good place to start doing these exercises. Most women have more strength than they realize, and they can very, very quickly see the results."

Kegel Balls and Barbells

Kegel balls and vaginal weights are designed for strengthening the pelvic floor. There are even Kegel barbells! All of these are designed to be used for vaginal weightlifting and are available from places like Dr. Barb DePree and Kim Anami's websites.

Pelvic Tone Vibrators

Pelvic tone vibrators are designed to restore pelvic muscle tone, strength, and control. They also provide clitoral and G-spot stimulation while stimulating and toning muscles with specially designed electrodes. Some models have a customizable shaft to fit different size vaginas. Many come with varying levels of muscle stimulation and vibration speeds. As the vagina gets toned and blood flow is increased, there will be more lubrication.

Clitoral Pump: Increase Sensation

Vacuum therapy is sometimes prescribed to increase circulation in the genital area for women. Clitoral pumps are specifically designed for this function and are used to increase blood flow to the clitoris, either before or between sexual encounters to help restore and increase clitoral sensation. Increased circulation offers the benefits of increased lubrication, sensation, and overall sexual satisfaction.

Laser Treatment for Vaginal Atrophy

According to Nicole Fleischmann, MD, there are vaginal laser treatments that can make a big difference and even reverse itchiness, dryness, pain, burning, and in some cases, even frequent urination.

The treatment Dr. Fleischmann uses is the MonaLisa Touch®. It's an in-office vaginal laser treatment that just takes a few minutes to perform once the vagina is treated with a topical cream to numb the tissue. This laser treatment stimulates production of collagen, to improve the functionality of the vagina and restore the proper trophic balance to the mucous membrane. After treatment, patients are advised to use ice packs to reduce swelling and a lubricant to keep things moist.

Dr. Fleischmann added that laser treatment doesn't always eradicate frequent urination or urinary incontinence, but has been effective in many cases.

She said, "I have women who have sexual relations into their seventies or eighties and they have no intention of giving that up. I try to help them keep that part of their life as long as they can. I've done a MonaLisa® on patients in their eighties and I've been shocked on how well it works on eighty-year-olds."

For women who cannot take estrogen supplements, the laser treatment could be a great alternative, according to Dr. Fleischmann. These women include those dealing with or who have dealt with breast cancer, or who had their ovaries removed and are in menopause.

In particular, breast cancer patients cannot take estrogen because estrogen feeds breast cancer tumors, so women with breast cancer are often taking medication to eradicate the estrogen in their bodies. Dr. Fleischmann said she is seeing women in their twenties and thirties diagnosed with breast cancer. These women are also candidates for laser treatment for vaginal issues.

Part Five

STOCK YOUR PANTRY FOR PLEASURE

These days, I keep it simple. I dubbed myself a "Wholefoodatarian," which means my meals are made from whole foods and are easy to prepare.

My go-to meal is a small portion of grass-fed meat, yam, avocado, and a big salad. Big salads are a staple in my house. Some of my favorite salad fixin's include baby romaine lettuce, beets, carrots, cilantro, cucumbers, olives, spinach, and tomatoes. In addition to grass-fed meat, fish, chicken, and a variety of beans and legumes are in the protein rotation. Most of the time my family eats what I eat. However, a couple of times a week I prepare dueling pastas—my family enjoys whole wheat pasta and I favor pastas made from beans and lentils. I recommend Modern Table Meals and Al Dente Gluten-Free Pasta.

In fall and winter, I enjoy making big pots of chili, soups, and stews. I select my produce based on the Dirty Dozen and the Clean Fifteen lists (see page 63). In the spring and summer, I add salads with quinoa, bean pasta, and a larger variety of veggies. I also LOVE summer fruit—I can live on cherries and watermelon! I love all of the recipes in this book and they are a part of the regular rotation.

Unlike my mother, I *love* spices and use them all the time, particularly garlic. Sautéed in Avohass Avocado Oil and served over veggies, in spaghetti sauces, and on brown rice and pasta. We are a pungent bunch! We are also a spicy bunch, which is why I always have Devil's Envy Spice in my pantry. It is a personal favorite! The creator, Michael Farca, shares on his site www .devilsenvyspice.com that he was raised by two immigrant parents (mother from Israel and father from Mexico) and both cultures have dynamic and flavorful cuisine. Michael explains, "We found plenty of products that hit spicy or flavor notes separately, but never together. Then one day, my aunt got an idea for a spicy, flavorful mix—and she nailed it! The results were both spicy and robust with flavor. It was the first batch of what we now call Devil's Envy."

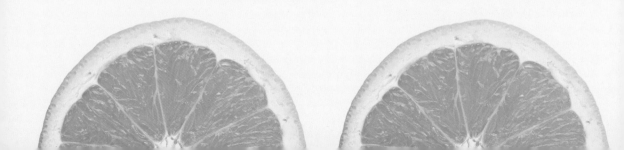

Chapter Thirteen

NUTS, BOLTS & BERRIES

We are down to the nuts and bolts of what to eat for optimal health. I look for foods that are organic, non-GMO, pesticide-free, local, and free-range. The following information is designed to help you select and prepare the freshest and healthiest ingredients.

USDA Certified Organic

The label "certified organic" verifies that the food was produced without the use genetic engineering, irradiation, or sewage sludge. Certified organic farms must adhere to ecological farming practices and are forbidden to use certain preservatives such as sulfites and nitrites.

Some produce is grown using the same organic standards but may not have undergone the expense and rigor of the USDA certification process. If I trust the source, and I do trust my local grocery market, I buy anything that is labeled "Organically Grown," whether it is USDA Organic Certified or not.

Organic Is Non-GMO

Certified organic food is guaranteed to be free of GMOs, genetically modified organisms.

Organic Is Not Guaranteed Pesticide-Free

Surprise! Organic produce is grown with pesticides. Organic pesticides, unlike the synthetic ones used on commercial agriculture, are made from natural sources. Unfortunately, there are still potential health risks associated with "natural pesticides." Fortunately, the Environmental Working Group (EWG) compiles a *Shopper's Guide to Pesticides in Produce* which provides information for consumers to reduce exposure to pesticides residues. You can sign up for a downloadable list at the EWG website.

Dirty Dozen and Clean Fifteen

The Dirty Dozen and Clean Fifteen are lists of produce that either consistently test high (dirty) or low (clean) for pesticide residue. I use these lists as a shopping guide to reduce my intake of pesticides in my diet. I only purchase produce on this list when it's labeled organic, or better yet, "pesticide-free." I buy conventional produce from the Clean Fifteen list unless the organic is on sale for the same or lower price.

The 2018 Dirty Dozen list includes: strawberries, spinach, nectarines, apples, grapes, peaches, cherries, pears, tomatoes, celery, potatoes, sweet bell peppers (honorable mention: lettuce and blueberries).

The 2018 Clean Fifteen list includes: avocados, sweet corn (organic & non-GMO!), pineapples, cabbage, onions, sweet frozen peas, papayas, asparagus, mangoes, eggplant, honeydew melon, kiwi, cantaloupes, cauliflower, and broccoli.

Animal Products

The healthiest animal products come from the healthiest and happiest animals. The healthiest animals have ample living quarters, access to the outdoors, are injected with neither hormones nor antibiotics, and eat a healthy diet. I always buy free-range chickens, free-range eggs, grass-fed/grass-finished meats, and wild salmon.

Jill Hillhouse, CNP, and Lisa Cantkier, CHN, authors and certified health nutritionists, share the following excerpts from their book, *The Paleo Diabetes Diet Solution,* to help decipher the healthy animal eating jargon.

Free-Range

"This label is used almost exclusively on poultry products, including eggs. The definition provided by the USDA states that producers must demonstrate that the poultry has been allowed access to the outside. While this sounds nice, it could just mean that there's a small door at one end of a very large barn that is open for a short amount of time each day and that very few birds, if any, actually make it outside. There are no standards as to how big the outdoor area is or whether it is concrete or pasture or bare ground."

Free-Run

"Free-run is not the same as free-range. While these birds are not in cages and are technically allowed to move around freely in the barns, the conditions are generally incredibly overcrowded. These birds do not have access to the outside."

Pasture-Raised

"This label generally applies to pigs and chickens, but could be found on all types of meat. The label implies that the animals lived primarily in fields or wooded areas, where they ate grass and other plants as well as bugs and insects. Grains might be added to the diet of pasture-raised animals during the winter, when pastures are covered with snow and the animals are brought inside. There is no legal or regulated definition of this term in the United States or Canada."

Grass-Fed

"Grass-fed applies to animals whose diet consists exclusively of grass for most of its life. This includes cow and sheep, not pigs and chickens. Grass-fed animals are usually pasture-raised, though grass-eating animals can also be fed hay in barns. Most food labeled grass-fed is from animals who spent most of their lives outdoors."

Grass-Finished

A product may say "grass-fed" on the packaging, but may have been "finished" on grain. This means the animal was fed grain, not grass or hay, during the last two or three months of its life. Beef from grass-fed cows is lower in calories and higher in Omega-3 fatty acids, vitamin E, and conjugated linoleic acid (CLA). When you can, select products labeled "100% grass-fed beef."

Wild or Farmed

Wild fish live in natural environments, have fewer calories, and a higher omega-3 content than farmed fish. Although both wild and farmed fish can contain pesticides, wild fish have them in lower concentrations. Farmed fish live in captivity which means they are most likely given antibiotics. Look for the "wild" label when purchasing fish.

Fresh and Local Produce

Nothing beats local for fresh produce (picked within the last forty-eight hours). If you are neither a farmer nor a gardener, then for you, fresh produce doesn't grow on trees. Fortunately, farmer's markets are an excellent source of fresh and local produce picked that same day.

Frozen, Packaged, and Canned

Frozen, and in some cases packaged, are the next best choices after fresh. Frozen fruits and vegetables are picked at their peak ripeness and quickly frozen to preserve their nutrients.

I keep a variety of frozen fruits at the ready for quick and nutritious smoothies.

Packaged produce is picked at its peak ripeness then pre-washed and cut and packaged. Air is removed to maintain freshness until the package is opened. I always check the expiration dates and make sure the bag is deflated, not puffed up like a balloon.

I buy canned beans. I love Amy's canned soups (great taste and the can's lining is BPA-free!). Other than mushrooms, I do not use canned vegetables; however, if you like them canned, go for it. The important thing is to eat your veggies!

Cooked or Raw: Preserve Key Nutrients

Once you have your fresh vittles, don't dilly-dally. It is best to consume, prepare, or preserve your produce within forty-eight hours, before it begins to spoil. Some foods are better for us when cooked, some when eaten raw. Here are some tips on how to prepare foods to maintain their most nutritional value.

Eat 'em Cooked, Eat 'em Raw

These vegetables will provide superior nutritional value when prepared as indicated in the following table: lightly steamed or roasted, eaten raw, or both! The nutritional punch of these foods is boosted when prepared with or paired with fat. Eat these vegetables with olive oil, avocado oil, avocados, nuts, seeds, or fatty fish.

Cooked	Raw	As you like
Asparagus	Apples	Broccoli
Carrots	Berries	Cabbage
Eggs	Bok choy	Cauliflower
Greens	Citrus	Garlic
Mushrooms	Cucumbers	Kale
Pumpkin	Lettuce	Onion
Spinach		Red peppers
Sweet potatoes		
Tomatoes		
Winter squash		
Zucchini		

Miscellaneous Clean Eating Tips

Here are other useful tips for preparing healthy meals.

- Steam, roast, braise, or pan-roast vegetables to a firm consistency ("al dente").
- Soak beans, nuts, and seeds prior to cooking or eating them raw.
- Purchase raw nuts (most roasted nuts are cooked in trans fat and vegetal oils).
- Pair iron-rich foods with vitamin C-rich foods to enhance iron bioavailability.
- Cook large quantities of food to eat throughout the week or freeze for later.
- Cook with oils that can withstand high temperatures: avocado oil, almond oil, hazelnut oil, and macadamia nut oil.

Designer Meals

The *Food Healing Nutrition Program* and *The Food Healing Kitchen Makeover* are two programs which include recipes individually tailored to your health concerns. Both were created by Susan Irby, CFNS, aka *The Bikini Chef®*, and Ward Bond, PhD, nutrition expert.

"The *Food Healing Nutrition Program* helps identify which specific nutrients may be lacking or which ingredients from foods in an individual diet are possibly harming to sexual function and vitality. *The Food Healing Kitchen Makeover* takes the foundation of the *Food Healing Nutrition Program* a step further by diving in to a six-week recipe-based program," shared Chef Irby.

Additionally, Erin Macdonald, RDN, and I will be offering *The Clean Eating Dirty Sex Total Makeover* to help readers implement the principles of this book. Check it out at www.cleaneating dirtysex.com.

Chapter Fourteen

THE CLEAN EATING DICTIONARY— ABC'S OF SEXUAL HEALTH

Here is a list of common ingredients included in the recipes along with a hint of information about their individual properties to enhance your sex life. This non-exhaustive list is intended to whet your appetite.

Almonds: provide essential fatty acids and zinc necessary for the production of sex hormones.

Apples: contain high levels of quercetin, an antioxidant flavonoid, which increases endurance.

Artichokes: long considered a natural aphrodisiac, increase the body's response to stimulation.

Asparagus: contains vitamins B6 and B9 which boost arousal, and vitamin E which stimulates the production of sex hormones.

Avocados: a healthy monounsaturated fat and a great source of energy.

Bananas: a carbohydrate, provide sustained energy and potassium to prevent muscle cramps.

Beets: have nitrates that the body converts into nitric oxide, increasing blood flow to all areas of the body.

Black Raspberries: packed with antioxidants and flavonoids which boost libido and stamina.

Blueberries: ("Blowberries") are antioxidant and anti-inflammatory and have special properties to alleviate ED.

Bone Broth: contains minerals to nourish the skin cells and calm inflammation in the body and encourages beneficial gut bacteria.

Carrots: provide muscle benefits, reduce ED, and help with fertility issues.

Cayenne: increases blood circulation, purifies and boosts the immune system, increases sex drive, and releases endorphins which produces feelings of euphoria.

Celery: contains two pheromones, androsterone and androstenol, which alter the scent in your sweat glands making men more attractive.

Chia Seeds: rich in Omega-3 fatty acids which increase blood flow by reducing inflammation in the arteries.

Chili Peppers: contain capsaicin, the compound that makes tabasco sauce hot, and increase heart rate and boosts metabolism.

Cinnamon: lowers blood sugar levels, increases libido and circulation, which is why it's a known aphrodisiac.

Dark Chocolate: from the cocoa bean, bursting with antioxidants and containing phenylethylamine, a chemical that boosts endorphins (feel-good hormones). It also contains flavonoids. I recommend chocolate with 70 percent cocoa (or higher), also known as dark chocolate.

Dates: a great source of iron. This aids female ovulation and increases sexual desire in both women and men. Medjool dates are particularly popular.

Figs: have long been associated with boosted fertility and that's because they contain magnesium and essential amino acids. Both are linked to sex hormone production and improved circulation.

Garlic: raw garlic, when crushed, produces the phytonutrient allicin which many believe increases blood flow to sexual organs. Eat it with your partner so your "garlic breaths" will cancel out.

Ginger: aids blood flow by improving arterial health which is important for sexual performance.

Grass-fed Beef: contains niacin (vitamin B3), a blood-flow booster, which may alleviate erectile dysfunction.

Kale: a superfood, high in magnesium and B vitamins which help support healthy levels of both female and male sex hormones. And it's packed with niacin (B3).

Kimchi: a staple in Korea, kimchi is made from fermented vegetables, and is a natural source of probiotics, the beneficial gut bacteria. (Note: some are made with fish sauce.)

Kombucha: a fermented black or green tea, packed with probiotics.

Maca: also known as natural Viagra®, known for its hormone-balancing and libido-enhancing properties. For more on maca, refer to Chapter Fifteen.

Nuts: a rich source of healthy fats that increase blood flow and help you feel full, great for a sexually enhanced diet, especially almonds, pecans, hazelnuts, macadamia, pistachio, pine, and walnuts.

Oats: (oatmeal) a healthy source of fiber, and a great source for l-arginine, an amino acid commonly used to treat erectile dysfunction.

Olives: according to an ancient Greek legend, green olives made a man more virile, and black olives increased desire in women. Green olives are heavy in vitamin E, while black olives have more iron.

Onions: the antioxidants in onions help increase a man's sperm count, a great plus if you're trying to conceive.

Oysters: well-known as aphrodisiacs due to their high zinc content, oysters can help balance sex hormones in men and women, and increase clitoral sensitivity in women.

Pomegranate: rich in antioxidants, which support blood flow and help alleviate erectile dysfunction.

Pumpkin Seeds: a healthy fat and a great source of zinc and magnesium, which boost testosterone levels.

Quinoa: a wonderful alternative to SAD carbs; a plant-based source of complete protein, and high in fiber, which helps keep hunger at bay.

Saffron: an excellent source of calcium, potassium, manganese, iron, selenium, zinc, and magnesium, and enhances sexual performance.

Sauerkraut: fermented cabbage, sauerkraut is a great source of natural probiotics essential for gut health.

Sesame Seeds: contain zinc, which aids in testosterone and sperm production in men. It's a great addition to the diet when trying to conceive.

Shrimp: high in iodine, used by the thyroid gland to regulate energy, and a great source of protein.

Spinach: high in arginine, an amino acid that metabolizes to nitric oxide, which helps initiate and maintain erections and enhances muscle growth.

Strawberries: ("Screwberries") are packed with B vitamins, promote heart health and circulation, increase sperm count, and have special properties to alleviate ED.

Sweet Potatoes: a delicious source of healthy carbs that doesn't spike blood sugar. They have beta-carotene and potassium, which provide muscle benefits and alleviate erectile dysfunction and fertility issues.

Tea: natural, herbal teas contain flavonoids which are great for increasing blood flow in both women and men.

Tuna: has protein and vitamin B12, which promotes nerve health, brain function, and red blood cells. All this means more energy and increased libido.

Water: essential for sexual health. Water hydrates the skin, increases metabolism up to 30 percent within an hour of drinking it, flushes toxins, pumps up the joints so they work better, and provides a number of other benefits.

Watermelon: heavy in l-citrulline, which relaxes the blood vessels allowing for increased blood flow, and has earned the reputation for being a natural Viagra®.

Wild Salmon: a great source of omega-3 fatty acids, which aid nitric oxide production, which helps maintain an erection.

Yogurt: widely known as a source of probiotics, yogurt helps balance gut health by promoting beneficial bacteria which in turn reduces inflammation and bloating, encourages weight loss, helps prevent yeast infections in women, and promotes balanced pH levels. Go for no sugar or low sugar varieties.

Chapter Fifteen

SEXUAL ENHANCEMENT SUPPLEMENTS

Ward Bond, PhD, nutrition expert, TV & radio host/producer, wrote the book, *Dr. Ward Bond's Natural Guide to Better Sex: How Pro-sexual nutrition can help you love better and longer.* The following are excerpts from that wonderful fact-filled book. Thanks, Dr. Bond, for sharing this information with my readers!

Dr. Bond shared, "My expertise lies in the field of nutrition. As you explore the suggestions and definitions in this book, you may be astounded at the great number of ways nutrition and supplements can enhance sexual satisfaction. One of the great revelations may be recognition that safe supplements can add so much to your own sexuality."

Arginine: an amino acid that increases the amount of nitric oxide in the blood. This improves erections in men and sensation for women. Arginine also increases sperm count.

Butcher's Broom: increases lower circulation (legs, genitals, feet). This should be used for impotence problems that are due to lack of circulation. Butcher's Broom works well in combination with Yohimbe, Arginine, and a number of other sexual-enhancement nutrients.

Catuaba: increases sexual potency and sexual desire and corrects impotence and other sexual dysfunctions in both men and women. It also improves mental alertness and memory.

Chrysin: a flavonoid which prevents the conversion of testosterone into estrogen. Chrysin has two major values: it encourages your body to produce more testosterone and prevents estrogenic side effects that often are tied to the use of prohormones such as the various Andros and DHEA.

DHEA: an abbreviation for dehydroepiandrosterone (pronounced dee-hi-dro-epp-ee-an-droster-own). It is a natural steroid and the most common hormone in our bodies. Produced by our adrenal glands, it is a precursor for the manufacturing of many other of the body's hormones—including sex hormones.

    Caution: DHEA is not recommended for those who have a history of breast, ovarian, uterine, or prostate cancers, since these are hormone-related cancers.

Ginkgo Biloba: improves blood flow and is beneficial in the treatment of erectile dysfunction. Ginkgo Biloba combines well with many different herbs that include circulation and aphrodisiac properties. Don't take ginkgo if you're on blood thinners; that caution includes a daily regimen of aspirin for heart health.

Histidine: an amino acid that creates histamine. Histamine is a useful aid to sexual arousal and also enhances orgasm. Histidine is used for increasing sexual pleasure and rekindling interest in sex. This supplement isn't recommended for people who are manic-depressive or schizophrenic, nor for those who take antihistamines. Avoid histamine if you have a severe allergic reaction to any of a number of foods or to bee stings.

Horny Goat Weed: its testosterone-like effect stimulates sexual activity in both men and women . . . stimulates the sensory nerves and, most significantly, increases sexual desire. It is also used to treat disorders of the kidneys, joints, liver, back and knees. It has anti-fatigue effects and helps prevent adrenal exhaustion.

Maca (Peruvian): a potato-like vegetable that grows in the mountains of Peru at elevations of 9,000 to 11,000 feet, making it the highest cultivated plant in the world. Undiscovered by the rest of the world until recently, maca has been a staple food of native Peruvians since before the time of the Incas, accepted in their world for both its nutritional and medicinal properties.

Maca is used to increase energy, stamina, and endurance and promote mental clarity. It contains a large number of essential amino acids and alkaloids which stimulate the reproductive system of both sexes. An interesting byway of this important finding is the fact that animals taken to the high mountains of Peru failed to reproduce ... until Maca was added to their diet.

Methionine: an amino acid, reduces the level of histamine in the body. High histamine levels can be a cause of premature ejaculation and over-excitability. Methionine works well when combined with schizandra for the treatment of premature ejaculation.

Mucuna pruriens: known by many common names, velvet bean, cowhage or cowitch, this plant indigenous to India is recognized as an aphrodisiac in the ancient practice of Ayurveda. It increases testosterone levels, leading to the addition of protein in the muscles and therefore increased muscle mass and strength. The extract is also known to enhance mental alertness and improve coordination. A clinical study confirmed the efficacy of mucuna pruriens seeds in the management of Parkinson's disease because of their L-dopa content.

Mucuna can cause irregular menstrual cycles in women of child-bearing age, so Mucuna is best saved for the menopausal phase of a woman's life cycle. For younger women, NADH may be the supplement of choice.

Muira Puama: an herb grown deep in the rainforest and commonly known as "Potency Wood." This is one of the best herbs for most men to use for erectile dysfunction, and it has an equally deserved reputation for increasing sexual desire. The shrub is native to Brazil and has long been used as a powerful aphrodisiac in South America. A recent clinical study has validated its safety and effectiveness in improving sex drive and sexual function in many patients.

Based on the many clinical reports documenting the libido and energy enhancing effects, Muira Puama increases free testosterone and/or suppresses excess estrogen.

NADH: a supplement that increases the level of dopamine in the brain which equates to increased sexual desire. Dopamine is a neurotransmitter responsible for strength, movement, coordination, alertness, memory function, mood, and sex drive. Dopamine seems to be an important aspect of sexual function, as dopamine improves libido, orgasm, and male ejaculation. Dopamine plays an indirect role in stimulating testosterone production. It also inhibits pituitary secretion of prolactin, high levels of which may interfere with the production of testosterone. Low dopamine levels have been linked with shyness, a finding with interesting implications for the relationship of the neurotransmitter to human socio-sexual interaction. Many women take NADH for energy, but find a very likeable side effect of sexual enhancement.

Saw Palmetto: an increasingly well-known herb that tones and strengthens the male reproductive system. It has been used as a boost to the male sex hormones. And it is a specific recommendation in cases of an enlarged prostate gland.

Saw palmetto may be beneficial for both sexes in balancing the hormones.

Women regularly use saw palmetto to stimulate breast enlargement and lactation as well as to treat ovarian and uterine irritability. It has been prescribed to aid reduced or absent sex drive, impotence, and frigidity. Saw palmetto also is used to increase vaginal wetness in females, and is quite effective when used in combination with wild oat.

Because of its potential hormonal effects, pregnant women should not use saw palmetto.

Schizandra: a small red berry-like fruit off a hardy vine of the magnolia family. Schizandra improves overall blood circulation, allowing heightened sensations in the female sex glands during intercourse.

It also helps to control premature ejaculation and prolong erection by lowering excessive histamine levels in the body.

Siberian Ginseng: one of the most popular and dependable supplements. It helps prevent impotence, enhances endurance stamina and sexual function, improves mental alertness, and relieves stress.

Ginseng root stimulates both physical and mental activity, improves endocrine gland function, and has a positive effect on the sex glands. This supplement is highly recommended if stress is the cause of one's impotence.

Tribulus terrestris: increases testosterone, luteinizing hormone (LH), follicle stimulating hormone (FSH), and estradiol. In men, this herb improves and prolongs the duration of erection. It exerts a stimulating effect on sperm by increasing the number of sperm, their motility, and their survival time. In women, increased sexual desire depends on the increases of testosterone and luteinizing hormone.

Tribulus increases sexual desire in those women who have had hysterectomies or ovariectomies. European research indicates this herb is used for ovarian sterility, neurasthenia (a condition of nervous exhaustion and physical tiredness that often follows depression), and menopausal depression.

One thing to remember when taking tribulus: It only works for eight weeks of continuous use. The brain realizes it has been tricked into producing more luteinizing hormone. So after eight weeks, discontinue use for 2–4 weeks and then resume.

Cautions:

- Tribulus should not be taken by pregnant women or children.

- It should not be taken by anyone with a psychosis, schizophrenia, or pheochromocytoma.
- Don't combine tribulus with any other psychoactive medication, such as tranquilizers, sedatives, stimulants (even over the counter decongestants like ephedrine), or antidepressants.

Tyrosine and Phenylalanine: amino acids involved in the creation of dopamine, a neurotransmitter associated with sexual behavior. It seems that higher levels of dopamine are associated with more sexual interest.

L-dopa is a chemical precursor of dopamine. The body uses L-dopa to make dopamine. You can increase your brain dopamine levels by taking tyrosine and phenylalanine or the herb mucuna pruriens and even NADH.

Increased brain dopamine activity caused by taking the drug L-dopa is believed to be the cause of a "hypersexuality" syndrome in people who take the drug for Parkinson's disease.

Wild Oat: known as avena sativa, wild oat stimulates both men and women quickly and effectively. In men it is quite effective for treating impotence and premature ejaculation. In women it increases sexual desire. Wild oat is an herb that has been shown to free up bound testosterone in both males and females, increasing both desire and performance.

It is also a nerve tonic, reported to strengthen the nervous system. That benefit also applies to sexual performance, because it could help in cases of impotence caused by stress and psychological problems.

Yohimbe Standardized Extract: (*Corynanthe yohimbe*), is an herb derived from the bark of the yohimbe tree found primarily in the West African nations of Cameroon, Gabon, and Zaire. The US Food and Drug Administration (FDA) approved Yohimbe as a treatment for impotence in the late 1980s. Since then it has been available as an over-the-counter dietary supplement, as well as a prescription drug.

Yohimbe dilates blood vessels and stimulates blood flow to the penis, causing an erection. It also acts on the central nervous system, specifically the lower spinal cord area where sexual signals are transmitted. Studies show Yohimbe is effective in 30–40% of men who suffer from impotence.

This supplement is primarily effective in men whose impotence is due to vascular, psychogenic, or diabetic problems. It usually doesn't work in men whose impotence is caused by organic nerve damage. In men without erectile dysfunction, yohimbe in some cases appears to increase sexual stamina and prolong erections.

Part Six

TURN-ON RECIPES

Now it's time to get into the kitchen, rattle some pots and pans, and cook up these clean meals to enhance your health! These fifty-nine sensual, delicious turn-on recipes—full of sexual-enhancing ingredients—are divided into five chapters: Breakfast in Bed, Erotic Entrees, Seductive Sides, Down and Dirty Desserts, and Sensual Smoothies and Milkshakes.

Unless otherwise stated, the recipes were created specifically for this book by the amazing Erin Macdonald, RDN. Erin and her cousin Tiffani Bachus, RDN, are the authors of *No Excuses! 50 Healthy Ways to ROCK Breakfast* and *No Excuses! 50 Healthy Ways to ROCK Lunch and Dinner*. They are the dietitians for *Clean Eating Magazine* and the founders of *U Rock Girl*. Their recipes can be found in *Clean Eating Magazine*'s Clean Eating Academy.

A special thanks goes out to Diana Stobo and Tess Masters for their recipe contributions. Diana Stobo is the award-winning author of the healthy lifestyle book *Get Naked Fast! Stripping Away the Foods That Weigh You Down* and Tess Masters is the author of *The Blender Girl* series.

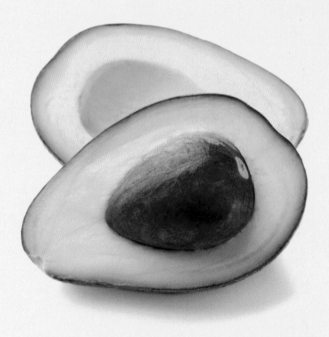

Chapter Sixteen

BREAKFAST IN BED

Rise and shine! Start your day with these delicious breakfast recipes, or if you prefer, these delicious breakfast recipes can be enjoyed any time.

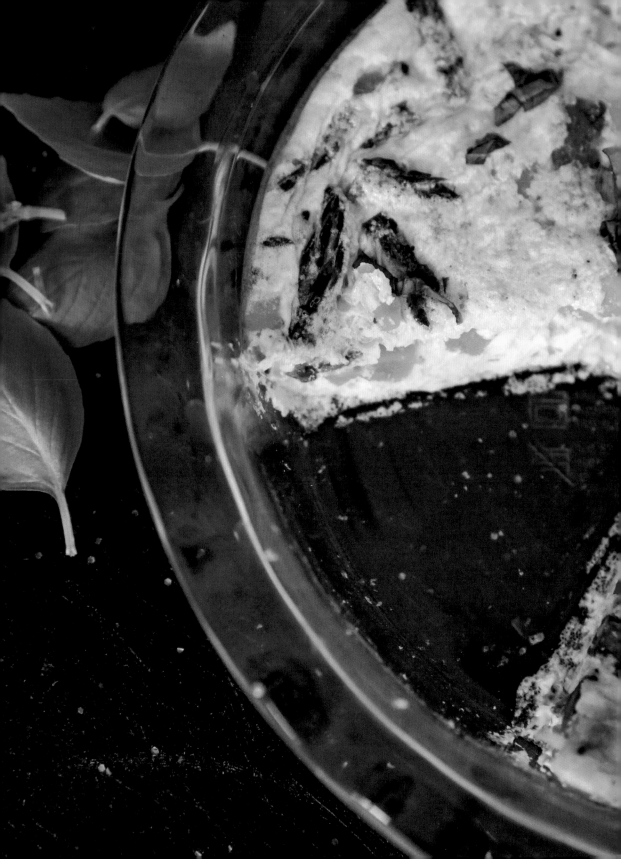

Asparagus, Leek, and Butternut Squash Frittata (SERVES 4)

Keen mental focus is enhanced by folate in asparagus. If you're thinking of conceiving, folate is also necessary for cognitive development of babies during pregnancy.

Ingredients

1 tablespoon plus 1 teaspoon avocado oil
1 leek, white part only, thinly sliced
1 cup diced butternut squash
Sea salt
Lemon pepper
5 spears of asparagus, woody ends trimmed, stalk chopped
6 eggs, whisked
½ tablespoon lemon zest
1 tablespoon lemon juice
Chopped basil for garnish

Directions

- Heat the oven to 365°F. Coat a pie plate with 1 teaspoon avocado oil. Set aside.
- Heat a large, nonstick skillet over medium-high heat and add remaining oil. When oil is hot, add the leeks and butternut squash with a pinch of salt and lemon pepper. Sauté for 5 minutes. Add the asparagus and sauté 1 minute. Pour into the pie plate.
- Whisk together the eggs, lemon zest, and lemon juice, and season with a pinch of salt and lemon pepper. Pour over the vegetables and place the dish into the oven to bake for 20 minutes. Remove to a cutting board and slice into wedges. Garnish with chopped basil.

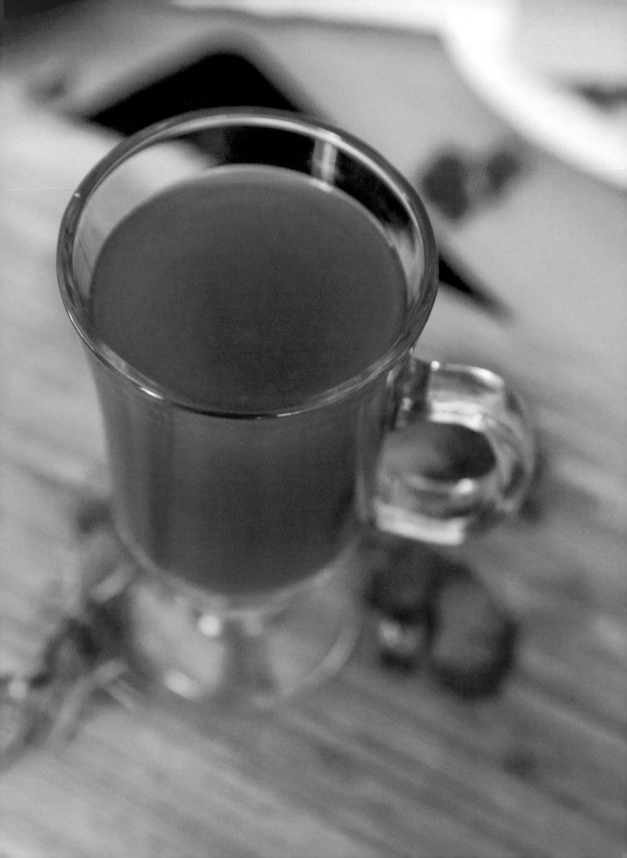

Beef Bone Broth (SERVES 10)

Grass-fed beef provides you with tons of niacin (vitamin B3) which is key in boosting libido and bedroom performance. Grass-fed beef is also higher in omega-3 fatty acids than corn-fed, preventing damage to your heart, and keeping it healthy for sex. And bone broth has collagen and gelatin which feeds the healthy bacteria in your gut and produces wonderful things for energy, blood flow, skin health, and so much more.

Ingredients

4 pounds marrow bones from grass-fed cows

1 pig's foot (your butcher can order these for you)

2 carrots, chopped

½ onion, chopped

2 garlic cloves

1 bay leaf

½ teaspoon sea salt

1 teaspoon pepper

2 tablespoons unfiltered apple cider vinegar

8–10 cups filtered water

Optional: plain gelatin powder packets

Directions

- Heat oven to 450°F. Place marrow bones on a sheet pan that's been covered with aluminum foil and place into the oven to roast for 30 minutes. Remove and transfer the bones into a large slow cooker (e.g. Crock-Pot).
- Add pig's foot, all vegetables, bay leaf, salt, pepper, apple cider vinegar, and water. Cover with lid and set slow cooker to the lowest heat setting for 12 hours or more. (Do not let this boil, because boiling destroys the gelatin in the pig's foot—so use low heat. If it's bubbling, then prop open the lid some to reduce the heat.) Add filtered water as necessary to keep the water level up.
- When done, strain through a fine mesh sieve into a container with a lid. Refrigerate overnight to allow fat to rise to the surface. Skim off fat. (Bone broth should have the consistency of Jell-O® when cold. If yours doesn't, you can warm the broth, then add plain gelatin packets you can buy in a powdered form at any grocery store. You'll have to experiment to see how many packets you need, but 2 is usually a good start.)
- Consume 1 cup of broth per day. Warm up before drinking.

Note: I know it sounds unappetizing, but you'll never taste the pig's foot and it adds a bunch of gelatin you need to make the broth effective. Gelatin comes from cartilage, so you may use bones that have cartilage, like a beef shoulder. Your butcher is a great source of suggestions for bones that have cartilage if you really don't want to use a pig's foot.

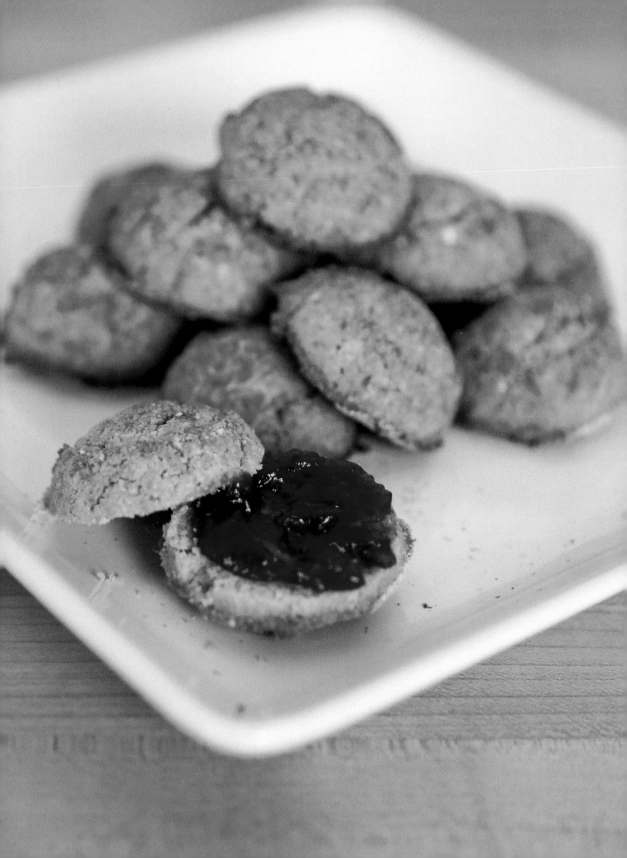

Better Body Biscuits (MAKES 14)

Many biscuits, muffins, and breakfast breads are loaded with refined sugars that cause blood glucose levels to spike, creating sex hormone imbalance. I encourage you to choose breakfasts higher in fiber and lower in refined sugar to help control blood sugar and maintain hormone balance—a benefit in the bedroom.

Ingredients

1½ tablespoons coconut flour (plus extra to flour the baking sheet)
1¾ cups almond flour
¼ teaspoon sea salt
½ teaspoon baking soda
¼ cup soft coconut oil
2 large eggs
2 tablespoons raw honey
2 tablespoons unsweetened almond milk

Directions

- Preheat oven to 350°F. Prepare a baking sheet with a non-stick Silpat silicone baking mat or parchment paper. Sprinkle a little coconut flour over the surface.
- Combine coconut flour, almond flour, salt, and baking soda in a large bowl. Whisk to combine.
- In another bowl, cream together the coconut oil, eggs, honey, and almond milk.
- Add flour mixture to the wet ingredients and stir until combined.
- Scoop out your biscuits onto the prepared baking sheet. You should get 14 small biscuits from this batter.
- Bake for 14 minutes. Serve with butter, pumpkin butter, or jam of your choice. Or slice them open and fill with wild smoked salmon and egg.

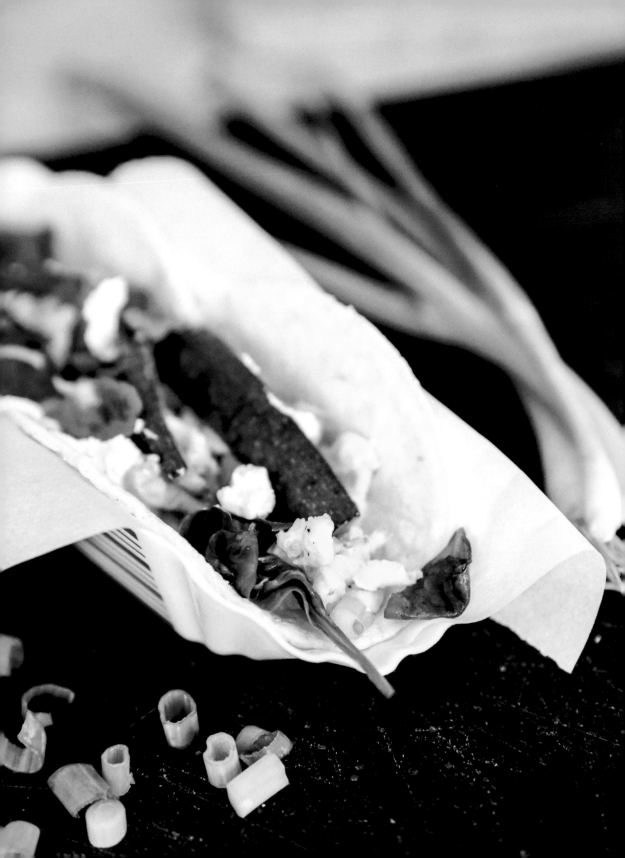

Breakfast Tacos (SERVES 1)

Storing up on B vitamins with the help of eggs allows for more calmness and can help men avoid premature ejaculation.

Ingredients

1 tablespoon avocado oil, divided
¼ cup chopped zucchini
1 green onion, sliced
1 cup organic baby spinach
2 eggs, whisked
2 organic corn tortillas
2 tablespoons salsa verde or salsa
    of choice
1 tablespoon cotija cheese
Chopped cilantro, for garnish

Directions

- Heat a nonstick skillet with ½ tablespoon avocado oil over medium-high heat until hot.
- Add the zucchini and cook 2 minutes. Add the green onion and spinach. Cook 1 minute. Add the remaining oil.
- When the oil is hot, add eggs and cook until set. Flip and cook until set.
- Heat corn tortillas on each side.
- Fill each warm tortilla with ½ of the egg mixture. Top with salsa verde and cheese. Garnish with chopped cilantro.

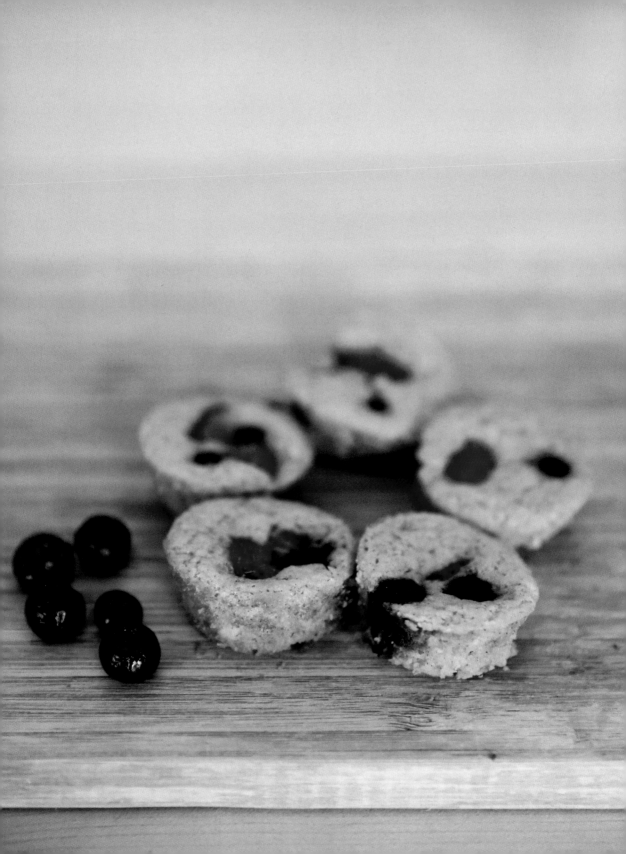

Lemon Berry Muffins (MAKES 12)

Replace the little blue pill (Viagra®) with blueberries! These little helpers relax blood vessels, improve circulation, and increase dopamine—resulting in a happy libido.

Ingredients

Coconut oil cooking spray
1 egg
1 tablespoon virgin coconut oil, melted
1 tablespoon coconut sugar
1 teaspoon lemon zest
1 tablespoon ground flax seed
½ cup unsweetened almond milk
½ cup almond flour
1 teaspoon baking powder
⅛ teaspoon sea salt
1 teaspoon pure vanilla extract
¼ teaspoon cinnamon
¼ cup fresh or frozen organic blueberries
¼ cup sliced fresh organic strawberries

Directions

- Heat oven to 350°F. Coat a mini muffin tin with coconut oil cooking spray.
- In a mixing bowl, whisk together egg, coconut oil, sugar, lemon zest, ground flax, and almond milk. Add the almond flour, baking powder, salt, vanilla, and cinnamon. Whisk until well blended.
- Fill each muffin opening about ⅔ full. Then add blueberries to half of the muffins and strawberries to the other half.
- Bake for 15 minutes. Remove and let cool before removing from the pan.

Overnight Oats (SERVES 1)

Forget boxed cereals. Oats are less refined than their O-shaped cousins, providing you with more beta-glucan. Cinnamon is one of those spices we like for female sexual health and banana provides important potassium and healthy carbs.

Ingredients

⅓ cup rolled oats
1 tablespoon ground flax seed
1 tablespoon chia seeds
½ teaspoon cinnamon
1 teaspoon pure vanilla extract
½ mashed banana
½ cup unsweetened almond milk
    or plain kefir
Toppings: fresh berries, chia seeds,
    additional cinnamon

Directions

- Mix everything (except toppings) together in a container and cover with a lid. Let it sit overnight in the refrigerator, then enjoy in the morning!

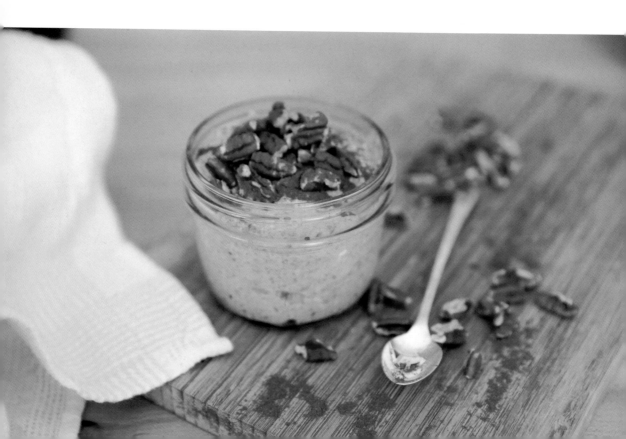

Rise and Shine Breakfast Bowl (SERVES 2)

Chicken-Apple sausage gives this dish a touch of sweetness plus the power of protein for increased energy.

Ingredients

⅓ cup quinoa, rinsed
1 tablespoon avocado oil
1 shallot, chopped
1 zucchini, chopped
2 cups cremini mushrooms, sliced
2 chicken-apple sausages, chopped
2 eggs (scrambled or sunny-side up)
Sea salt
Cracked lemon pepper
Baby greens, for garnish

Directions

- Place quinoa in a pot with ⅔ cup water and cover with lid. Bring to a boil and reduce heat to a simmer, cooking for 13 minutes or until quinoa is fluffy.
- Place a large nonstick skillet over medium-high heat and add the oil. When hot, add the shallot, zucchini, and mushrooms, and sauté for 5 minutes. Add the chopped sausage and cook 2 minutes more.
- Cook the eggs as you desire. It's your choice if you want to make them sunny-side up (so you can have a runny yolk to coat everything) or scrambled.
- To assemble the bowls: place half the quinoa in each of 2 bowls. Divide vegetable-sausage mixture on top of the quinoa. Top with egg. Season with some sea salt and cracked lemon pepper. Garnish with baby greens.

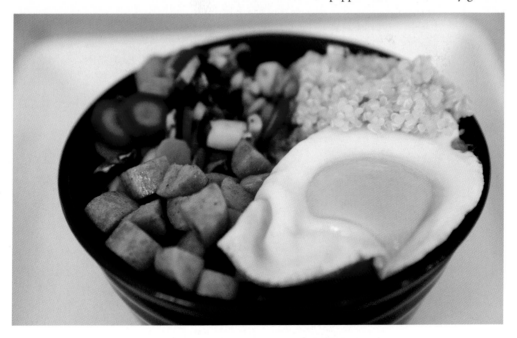

Southwest Frittata (SERVES 2)

Avocado oil is a healthy fat to keep you satiated and help with blood flow, and the eggs add protein to build strong muscles.

Ingredients

1 tablespoon avocado oil
¼ cup chopped sweet yellow onion
¼ cup chopped roasted red pepper
4 eggs, whisked
½ teaspoon ground cumin
Juice of ½ lemon
¼ teaspoon cracked lemon pepper
2 tablespoons chopped cilantro
2 tablespoons crumbled queso
    fresco
¼ teaspoon chili paste or red
    pepper flakes

Directions

- Heat oven to broil.
- Place a medium nonstick pan on the stove over medium-high heat and add the avocado oil. When hot, add the onion and roasted red pepper and sauté for 3 minutes.
- Whisk together the eggs, cumin, lemon juice, lemon pepper, cilantro, queso fresco, and red pepper flakes in a bowl. Add to the pan and lower the heat on the stove to medium. Let the bottom set on the eggs, cooking about 4 minutes. Transfer to the oven and broil for 2 minutes or until the top is set and lightly golden.

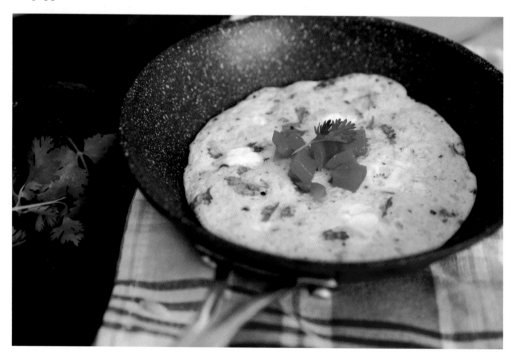

Sweet Potato Toast   (SERVES 2)

This recipe includes wild salmon which helps men with staying power, as it increases the production of nitric oxide, the building blocks of the male erection. And anything made with red chili peppers, like red pepper flakes or chili paste, is known to help with blood flow, another boost to staying power.

Ingredients

Virgin coconut oil or avocado oil
1 large sweet potato (orange flesh),
    cut on the diagonal into ½-inch
    planks
Cracked lemon pepper
2 slices wild smoked salmon or
    wild lox
2 large eggs
1 small avocado, peeled
½ cup cilantro
Juice of ½ lemon

Directions

- Heat a large nonstick skillet over medium-high heat and add 1 tablespoon coconut or avocado oil. When hot, add the sweet potato planks. Season with lemon pepper. Cook 2 minutes (or until golden on the bottom); flip and cook another 2 minutes. Remove to a platter. Top each sweet potato plank with a slice of wild smoked salmon.
- Return the skillet to the stove and coat with a splash of oil. When hot, crack eggs, leaving a little space between them. Season with lemon pepper. Cook 1–2 minutes and then flip each one, cooking another 1–2 minutes, depending on desired yolk firmness. Place eggs on top of wild smoked salmon.
- In a blender or small food processor, puree the avocado, cilantro, and lemon juice. Drizzle over the eggs.

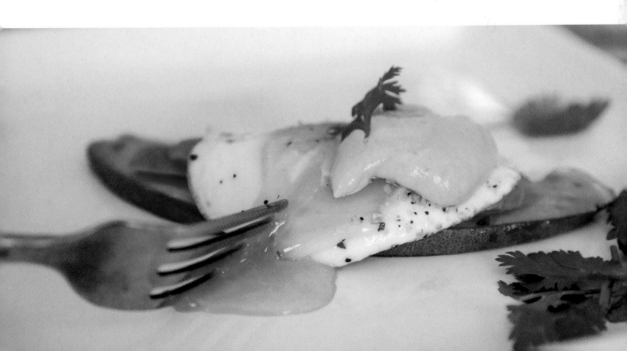

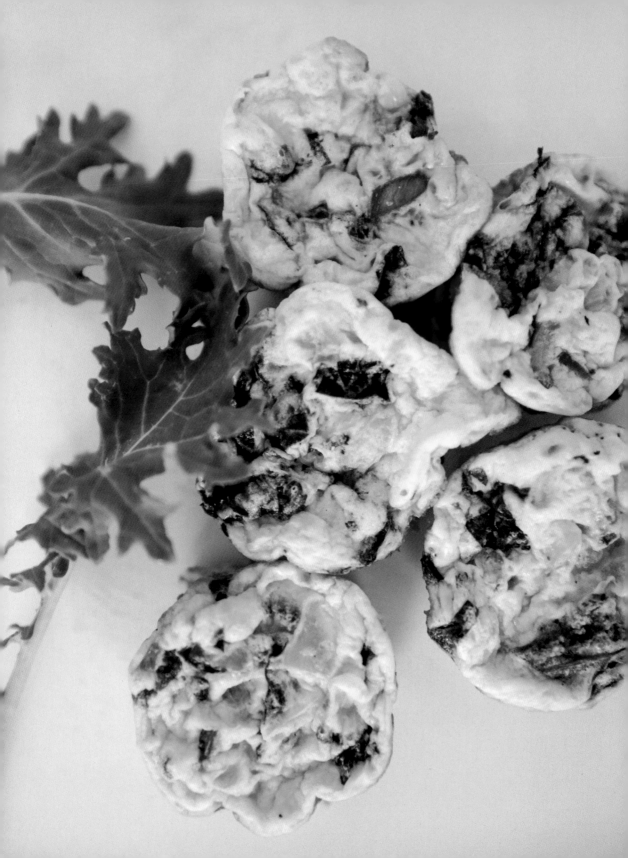

Veggie-Filled Egg Muffins

Want to spice up your sex life without spicy foods? Onions (like all spicy foods) have been found to boost libido and sex drive.

Ingredients

1 tablespoon avocado oil
½ sweet yellow onion, chopped
1 cup chopped mushrooms
Sea salt
Lemon pepper
2 cups organic baby spinach leaves
6 eggs, whisked
2 tablespoons parmesan cheese
*Optional: add a little heat by
  adding ¼ teaspoon chili paste
  or red pepper flakes to the
  whisked eggs

Directions

- Heat oven to 350°F. Prepare a 12-cup muffin tin by coating the inside of each opening with a bit of avocado oil.
- Place a large nonstick skillet over medium high heat and add avocado oil. When hot, add the onion and mushrooms, a pinch of salt, and a generous sprinkle of lemon pepper. Sauté 4 minutes. Add the baby spinach and cook 1 minute, or until wilted. Transfer vegetables to the muffin tin, filling each evenly, about ½–⅔ full.
- Whisk together eggs, parmesan cheese, and ½ teaspoon lemon pepper. Pour eggs evenly over the vegetables. Place muffin tin into the oven and bake for 18 minutes. They will puff up when they cook and fall once they are taken out of the oven.

Note: 2 muffins = 1 serving. Once they are cool, you can place them into zip-top bags and store in the freezer for future use.

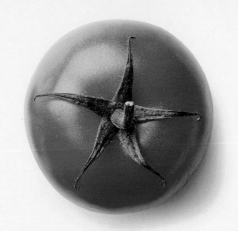

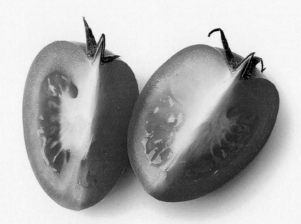

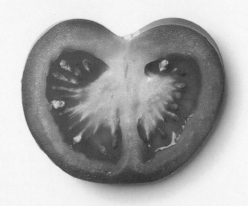

Chapter Seventeen

EROTIC ENTREES

For your big meals, here are some erotic entrees that incorporate the clean-eating, sex-enhancing foods we've discussed throughout the book.

Body Bowl

(SERVES 2)

Greeks have long believed that carrots were the secret to great sex, possibly providing those who partake with increased libido and bedroom wisdom.

Ingredients

1 carrot, shredded
½ cucumber, peeled and diced
½ cup cooked quinoa
⅔ cup black beans
½ mango, diced
1 avocado, diced
1 tablespoon chopped cilantro
2 tablespoons salsa verde

Directions

- Mix everything together and enjoy!

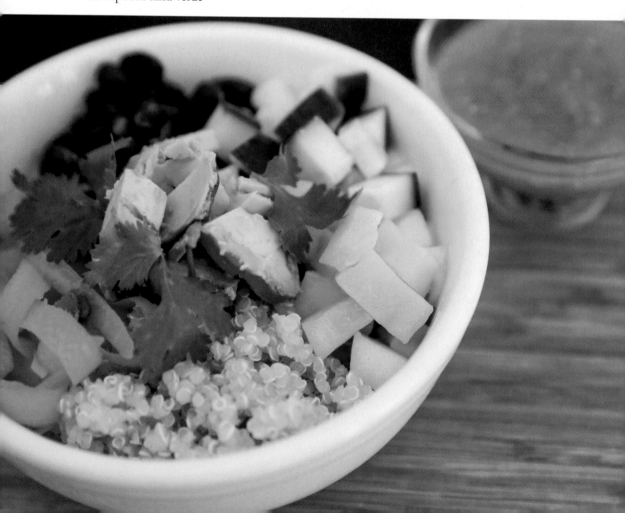

Chicken and Vegetable Soup (SERVES 10)

Egyptians have been using garlic to increase stamina for thousands of years. Put that to the test tonight!

Ingredients

1 whole organic chicken
½ sweet yellow onion, chopped
2 carrots, peeled and chopped
2 garlic cloves
1 (½-inch) piece ginger
3–4 sprigs fresh thyme
2 sprigs fresh rosemary
8 cups filtered water
1 teaspoon sea salt
1 teaspoon cracked lemon pepper
2 tablespoons apple cider vinegar
2 tablespoons yellow miso paste

Directions

- Wash chicken and place in a slow cooker. Add all remaining ingredients. Cover with lid and cook on the lowest heat setting for at least 8 hours (simmer, not boil).
- When done, remove the chicken (it will fall apart when you take it out) to a large plate and let cool for a few minutes. Separate the meat from the skin and bones and return the meat to the slow cooker. Discard the skin and bones, or save for bone broth.
- Stir the soup and taste. Add more salt and pepper if desired.

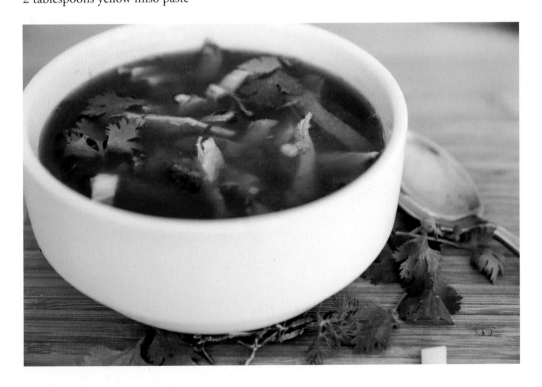

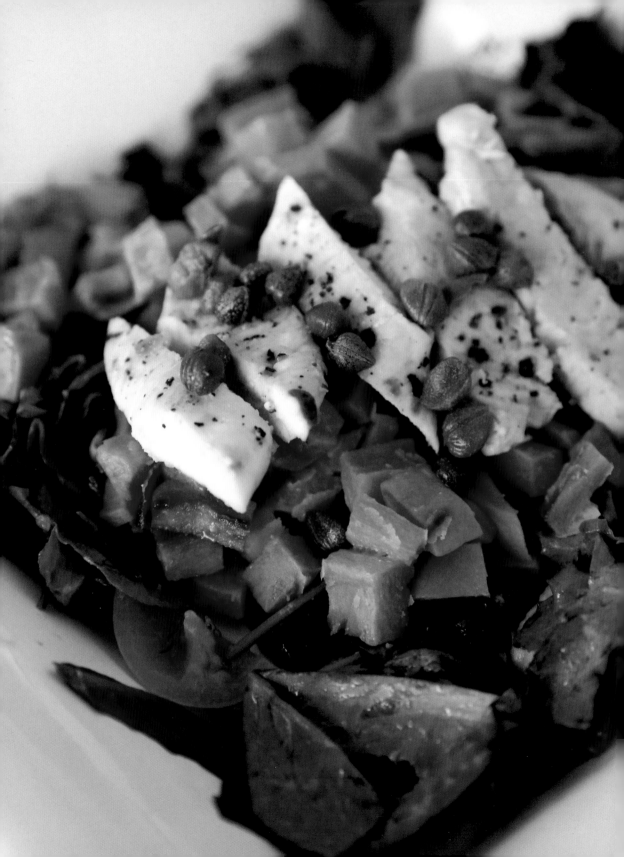

Chicken Scallopini with Lemon Caper Sauce (SERVES 2)

Keep your brain sharp, witty, and charming with the neurological benefits of vitamin B12, found in chicken. And keep your blood flow up with the healthy fats found in avocado oil.

Ingredients

2 tablespoons avocado oil, divided
Zest of ½ lemon
1 tablespoon lemon juice
1 teaspoon Dijon mustard
⅛ teaspoon sea salt
⅛ teaspoon cracked lemon pepper
2 chicken breast cutlets
1 tablespoon capers

Directions

- Make the lemon sauce: place 1 tablespoon avocado oil, lemon zest, lemon juice, mustard, salt, and pepper in a small container with a lid. Cover and shake until well blended and creamy. Set aside.
- Heat 1 tablespoon avocado oil in a large nonstick pan over medium high heat. When hot, add the chicken and season with a pinch of salt and pepper. Let cook 3 minutes, or until golden on the bottom. Flip and let cook for 2 minutes. Cover the chicken with the sauce and add the capers to the pan. Let cook 2 minutes.
- Serving suggestion: remove to a plate and serve with quinoa and garlicky greens.

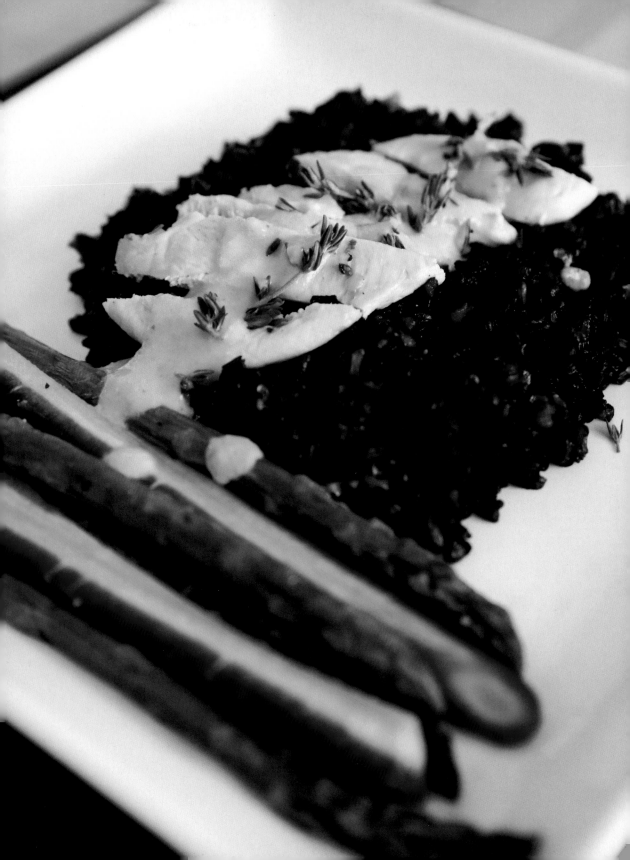

Chicken with Lemon Hummus Sauce (SERVES 2)

Baking eliminates the trans fats often found in fried chicken, which kill male libido.

Ingredients

1 tablespoon avocado oil
8 ounces chicken breast tenders
¼ teaspoon cumin
¼ teaspoon garlic powder
Pinch of cracked lemon pepper
Pinch of sea salt
4 cups baby arugula
2 tablespoons hummus (whatever flavor you like)
Juice of ½ lemon
2 tablespoons pine nuts (or any nut you like)
2 tablespoons dried cranberries (or organic cherries or apricots)

Directions

- Heat the oil in a large nonstick pan over medium-high heat. When hot, add the chicken and season it with cumin, garlic powder, lemon pepper, and salt. Let cook 8–10 minutes, or until the bottom is golden. Flip and cook an additional 8–10 minutes.
- Place arugula on a dinner plate. Top with the chicken. Mix the hummus with the lemon juice and spoon on top of the chicken. Sprinkle with pine nuts and dried cranberries.

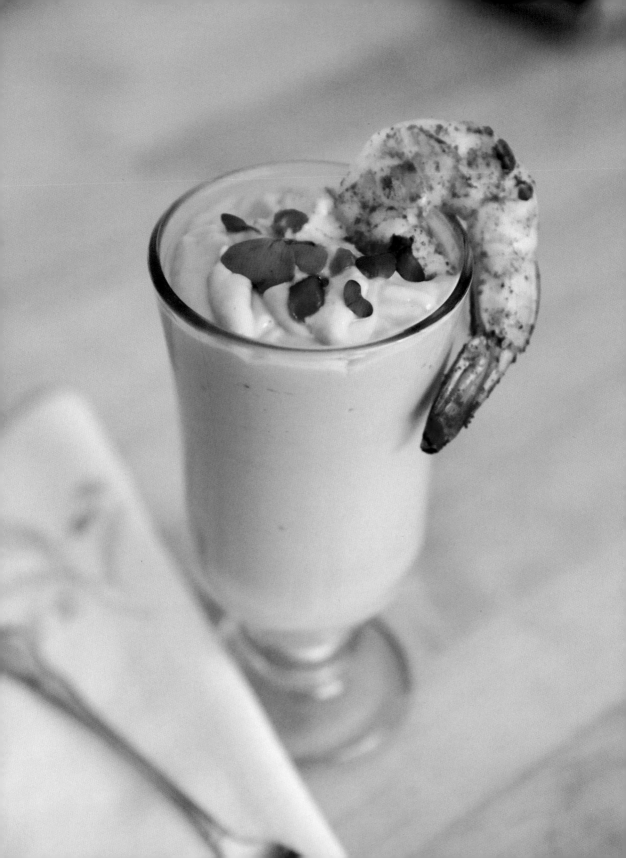

Chilled Cucumber Avocado Soup with Spiced Shrimp *(SERVES 4)*

Spice up the moment with roasted red pepper flakes, which increase your heart rate, turn up your libido, and heighten your arousal.

Ingredients

1 large hothouse or English cucumber, peeled, seeded, and coarsely chopped
2 large avocados, pitted, peeled, and quartered
1½ cups plain kefir or buttermilk
2 tablespoons red wine vinegar
1 teaspoon coconut sugar
Juice of 1 lime
Sea salt

Topping Ingredients

Roasted red pepper
Pea shoots
Optional: cold crab or sautéed shrimp

Directions

- Place cucumber, avocados, kefir or buttermilk, vinegar, coconut sugar, lime juice, and salt in a blender and blend until smooth. Taste and add more salt if needed.
- Pour into bowls and garnish with chopped roasted red pepper and pea shoots.

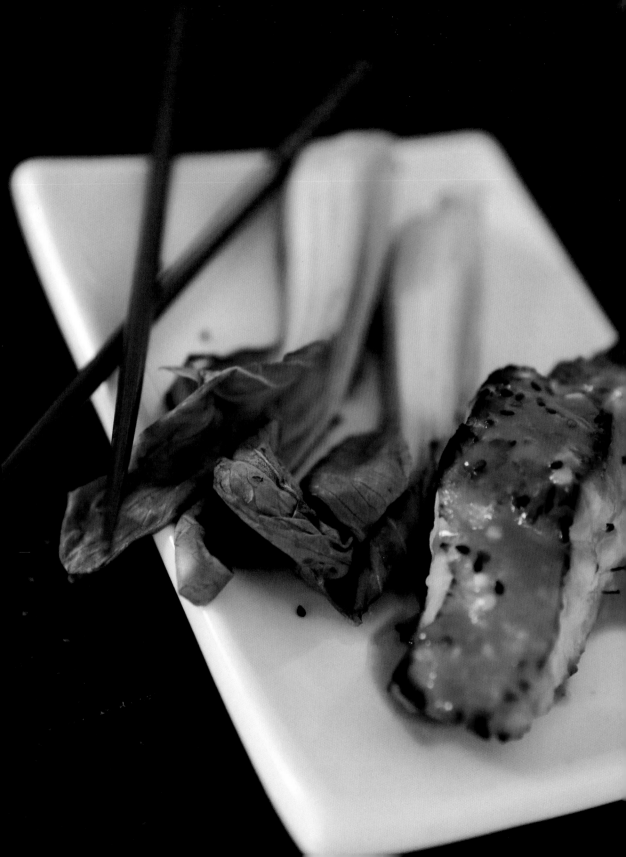

Miso-Glazed Black Cod with Baby Bok Choy (SERVES 2)

Sesame seeds have been linked to increased testosterone. Healthy testosterone levels are important for both men and women and in turn improve sexual health.

Ingredients

1 tablespoon sweet white or yellow miso paste
1 tablespoon low-sodium tamari or soy sauce
1 teaspoon sesame oil, divided
1 teaspoon rice vinegar
10 ounces black cod (also known as sablefish, or you may substitute Chilean sea bass), cut into two portions
3 baby bok choy, halved
1 teaspoon black or white sesame seeds

Directions

- Line a baking sheet with aluminum foil and set aside. Place a rack on top of the baking sheet. If you have 2 racks inside the oven, place one rack about 4–6 inches below the heating element and the other one in the middle level of the oven. Set oven to broil.
- In a bowl, mix together the miso, tamari, ½ teaspoon sesame oil, and vinegar until smooth for a marinade. Place the fish in a zip-top bag, pour the marinade over the fish, and let it marinate for 30 minutes.
- Remove the fish from the bag and place on the hot baking sheet. Place the baking sheet on the top rack of the oven and broil 4 minutes. Flip and broil another 4 minutes. Then move the fish to the middle rack and cook 2 minutes more. Flip and cook an additional 2 minutes.
- While the fish is cooking, add additional sesame oil (½ teaspoon) into a skillet over medium-high heat. When hot, add the baby bok choy and cook 2 minutes. Flip and cook another 2 minutes.
- Transfer the bok choy and the fish to two serving plates and garnish with sesame seeds.

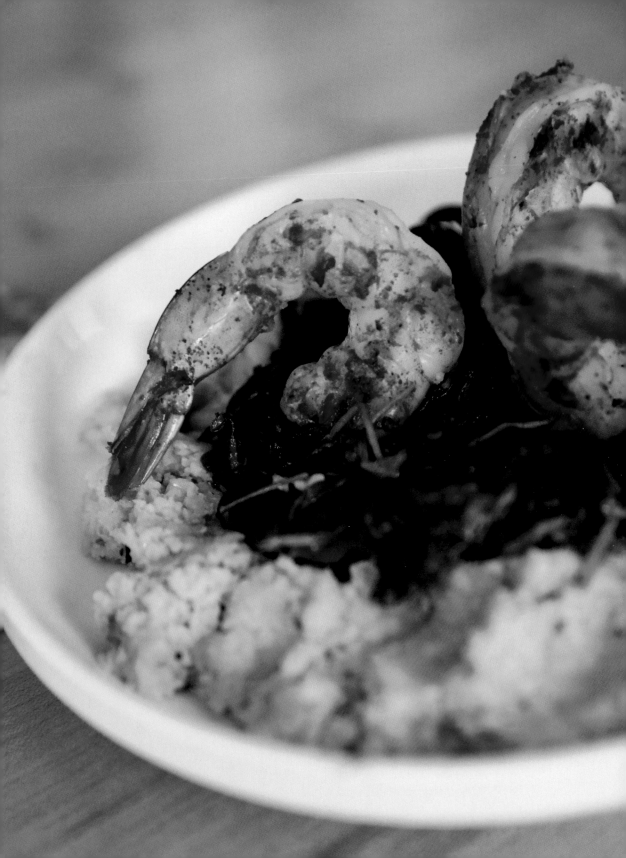

Shrimp with Cauliflower Mash and Garlic Kale (SERVES 4)

Shrimp are high in iodine, which is used by the thyroid to keep you energized.

Cauliflower Mash Ingredients

1 head cauliflower, broken into florets

Sea salt

Cracked black pepper

5 cloves garlic

2 tablespoons parmesan cheese

½ cup low-sodium vegetable broth (divided, quantity will vary)

Garlic Kale Ingredients

1 tablespoon coconut oil

3 garlic cloves, minced

3 cups baby kale (or any baby greens you like), chopped

Zest plus juice of 1 lemon

Sautéed Shrimp Ingredients

1 tablespoon coconut oil

1–1½ lbs. shrimp, peeled and deveined

½ teaspoon each chili powder, garlic powder, smoked paprika

Sea salt and black pepper

Directions

- Preheat oven to 375°F. Line a baking sheet with aluminum foil and coat with cooking spray. Place cauliflower on baking sheet and season with salt and pepper. Wrap the garlic cloves in foil and place on same baking sheet. Place in oven and roast 30 minutes or until cauliflower is lightly golden. Remove and let cool 5 minutes.
- Place cauliflower and garlic in food processor and puree with parmesan cheese and ¼ cup vegetable broth. Add more broth if too thick. You want the consistency of mashed potatoes. Season to taste with sea salt and pepper.
- Heat a large sauté pan over medium-high heat and add coconut oil. When hot, add the garlic and kale and sauté 5 minutes. Sprinkle with lemon zest and lemon juice. Remove from pan.
- Heat pan over medium-high heat with coconut oil. Toss the shrimp with the spices and then place in the hot pan. Cook 2 minutes per side. Remove to a plate and serve with garlic kale and the cauliflower mash.

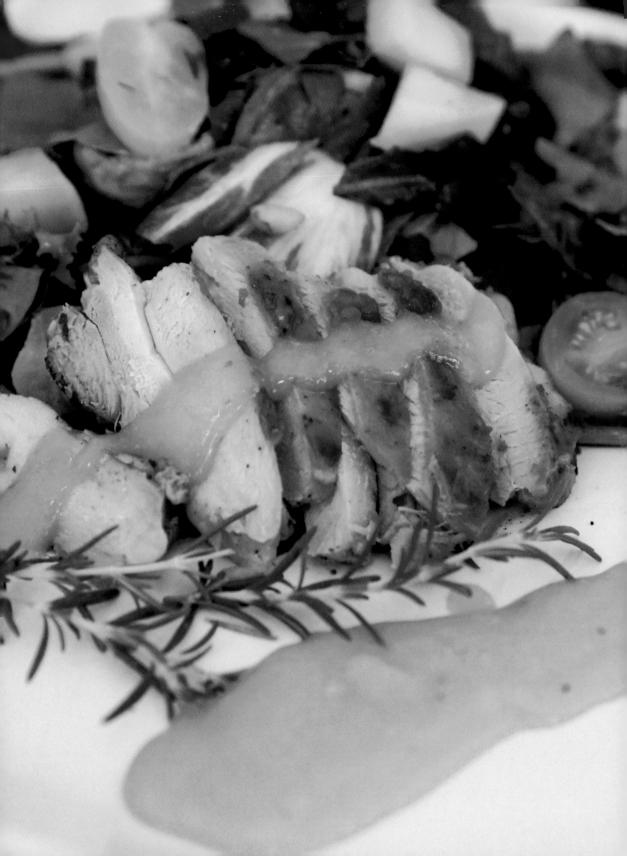

Spiced Chicken Thighs (SERVES 4)

Chicken thighs are high in B vitamins that are necessary for turning your calories into energy to keep you going through the night.

Ingredients

½ teaspoon smoked paprika
½ teaspoon ground cumin
½ teaspoon garlic powder
½ teaspoon onion powder
½ teaspoon cracked lemon pepper
½ teaspoon pink Himalayan sea
   salt
1 tablespoon coconut oil
4 boneless, skinless organic
   chicken thighs

Directions

- Combine all spices in a bowl and stir well.
- Heat the oil in a large nonstick pan over medium-high heat. When hot, add the chicken and season with half of the spice mix. Cook 5 minutes or until golden on the bottom. Flip and season with remaining spice mix.
- Cover the pan with a lid and cook 5–6 minutes or until the other side of the chicken is golden and the chicken is cooked through. You may serve the chicken with a salad, as shown in the photograph.

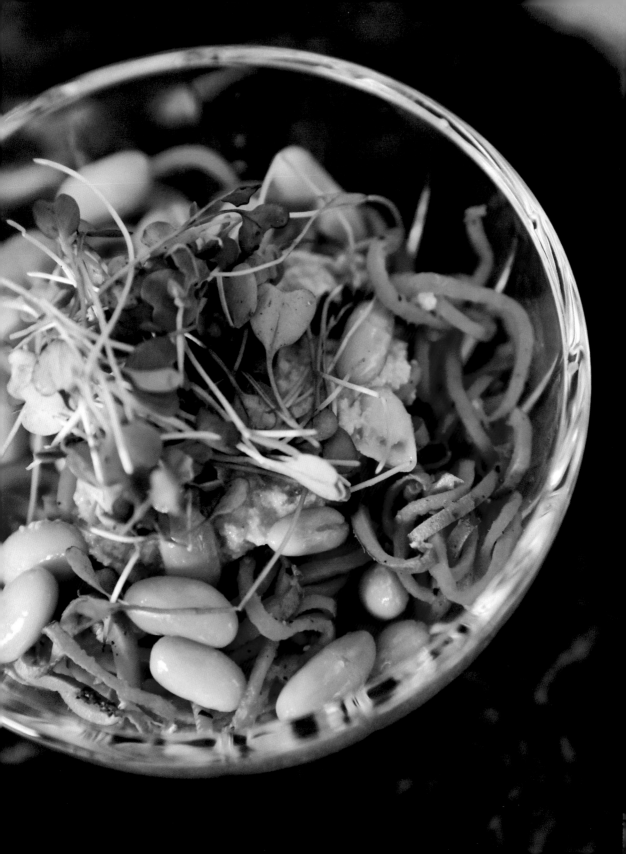

Sweet Potato Noodles with Garlic White Beans and Harissa Sauce (SERVES 4)

The beta-carotene in sweet potatoes improves the count and quality of the sperm in men.

Ingredients

1 cup raw cashews, soaked in water for at least 4 hours

1 tablespoon harissa (a Moroccan spice like chili pepper paste)

1 tablespoon plus 1 teaspoon coconut oil

1 sweet potato, peeled and spiralized (you can also find these already spiralized at some grocery stores)

1 can white cannellini beans, rinsed and drained

2 cloves garlic, minced

Sea salt

Lemon pepper

1/3 cup microgreens

Directions

- Drain the cashews and place in a blender or food processor. Pulse to break down the nuts and add 1 tablespoon water at a time to create a medium-thick creamy consistency. Add 1 tablespoon harissa to the cashew cream.
- Heat 1 tablespoon coconut oil in a large pan. When hot, add the sweet potato spirals. Cook for 5 minutes. Remove to a plate and sprinkle with sea salt.
- Heat 1 teaspoon coconut oil in pan over medium heat. When hot, add the beans and garlic. Cook 2–3 minutes. Season with salt and lemon pepper. Remove from heat.
- To assemble bowls, place sweet potato in bowl and drizzle harissa cashew cream on top. Place a scoop of garlic beans on top of noodles and then garnish with microgreens.

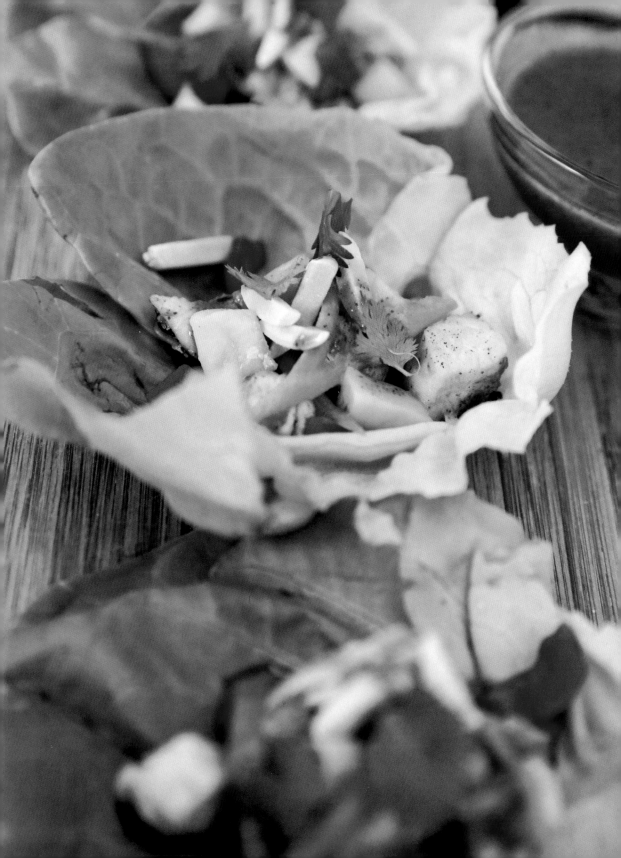

Thai Chicken Tacos with Peanut Sauce (Lettuce Wrapped)

(SERVES 4)

Get a little spicy by adding ginger into your diet! It improves heart health, helps clear arteries, and improves circulation.

Peanut Sauce Ingredients

2 tablespoons organic peanut butter (may substitute almond or cashew butter)
2 tablespoons low-sodium tamari or soy sauce
2 tablespoons grated ginger
1 tablespoon sesame oil
2 tablespoons raw honey
⅛ teaspoon Devil's Envy Red Pepper Spice
½ lime, juiced

Marinade Ingredients

½ cup orange juice
¼ cup low-sodium tamari or soy sauce
2 tablespoons raw honey
1 tablespoon grated ginger
½ lime, juiced
¼ teaspoon red pepper flakes

Taco Filling Ingredients

2 organic chicken breasts
Butter lettuce leaves
2 carrots, shredded or julienned
1 red bell pepper, sliced thin
1 cup shredded Napa cabbage
½ mango, peeled and chopped
2 tablespoons chopped peanuts
2 tablespoons fresh cilantro leaves
¼ cup bean sprouts

Directions

- To prepare the peanut sauce, pour all ingredients into a bowl and whisk until blended.
- To prepare the marinade, pour all the ingredients into a large zip-top bag.
- Cut chicken into 1-inch pieces and place in the bag with the marinade and seal for at least 1 hour.
- Coat a large nonstick pan with cooking spray and place over medium-high heat. When hot, add the chicken and cook about 2–3 minutes per side.
- Place 2 large butter lettuce leaves on each plate. Add ½ cup chicken pieces, some of the carrots, red pepper, cabbage, and mango.
- Pour some of the peanut sauce over the top and garnish with some chopped peanuts, cilantro, and bean sprouts.

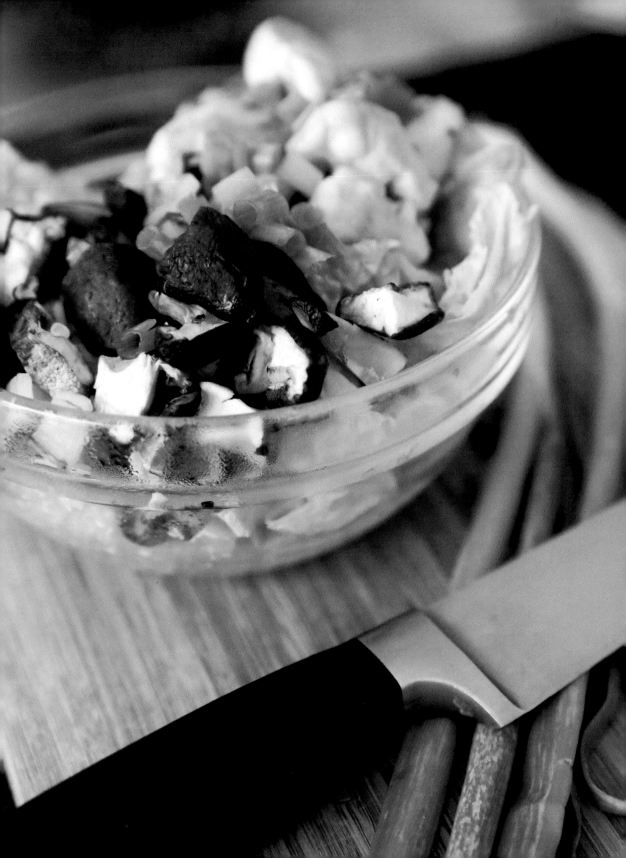

Umami Chicken and Mushroom Bowl with Dijon Citrus Dressing (Serves 2)

Quinoa will keep your stomach fuller longer with complete proteins and lots of fiber. And the dressing has citrus fruits, vitamin C powerhouses, to boost your immune system to keep you out of bed during the day and in bed at night.

Dijon-Citrus Dressing Ingredients

2 tablespoons rice vinegar
1 tablespoon whole grain Dijon
   mustard
1 tablespoon low-sodium tamari
2 teaspoons lime juice
½ teaspoon orange zest
2 teaspoons orange juice
½ teaspoon fish sauce
½ teaspoon toasted sesame oil

Umami Chicken and Mushroom Bowl Ingredients

5 shiitake mushrooms
½ shallot, chopped
½ cup cooked quinoa
½ cup shredded Napa cabbage
½ cup bean sprouts
1 green onion, chopped
1 large, organic chicken breast,
   cooked and shredded

Directions

- Place all dressing ingredients into a mason jar (or other glass container with a lid) and screw on the lid. Shake vigorously.
- Coat a nonstick skillet and place over medium high heat. When hot, add the mushrooms and shallot and sauté until soft, about 4–5 minutes. Remove to a plate to cool.
- Fill each bowl with quinoa, cabbage, bean sprouts, and green onion. Top with the cooled mushroom mixture and shredded chicken. Pour the Dijon dressing over the bowls. Mix and enjoy.

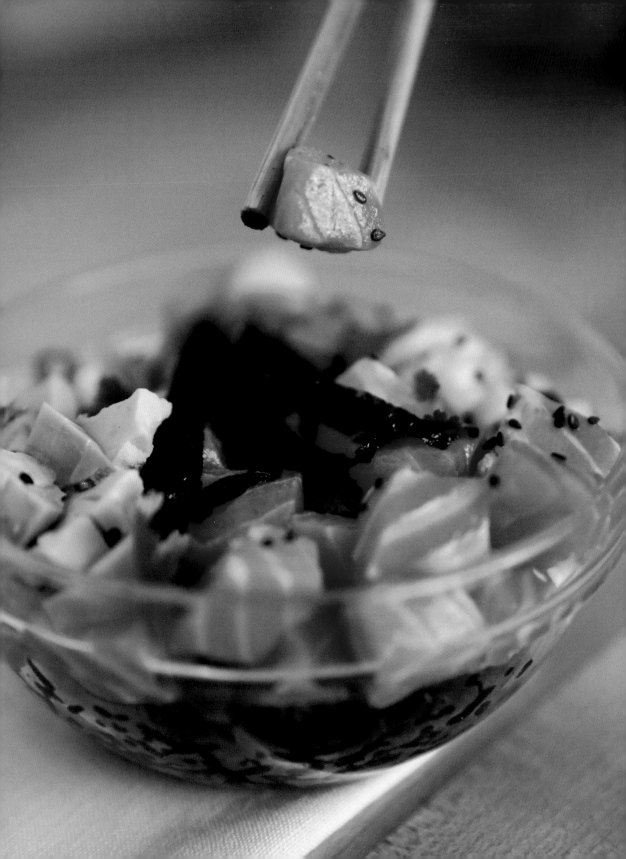

Wild Salmon Poke Bowl (SERVES 2)

Get wild with salmon and benefit from reduced erectile dysfunction and increased nitric oxide production, helping you both be ready.

Ingredients

½ cup black rice
1 cup water
8 ounces sashimi-grade wild
    salmon or ahi tuna
1 tablespoon low-sodium tamari
1 tablespoon seasoned rice vinegar
½ teaspoon toasted sesame oil
1 hothouse cucumber, peeled and
    diced
3 rainbow carrots, peeled and
    sliced into thin rounds
2 green onions, thinly sliced
½ tablespoon sesame seeds, toasted
1 avocado, cubed
Cilantro, for garnish
1 sheet of seaweed snack, sliced
    into thin strips for garnish

Directions

- Place rice and 1 cup water into a saucepan. Cover pan and bring to a boil, then reduce to a simmer, and cook about 25 minutes or until all the liquid has been absorbed. Remove and let cool.
- Slice fish into 1-inch pieces and then chop into ½-inch squares (the size of dice). Place in a large mixing bowl.
- Combine half the tamari, half the rice vinegar, and sesame oil, and then pour over the fish. Toss to coat and let marinate for 10 minutes.
- Place the cucumber, carrot, green onions, and sesame seeds in a bowl and top with remaining tamari and rice vinegar.
- Place a scoop of cooked and cooled rice in the bottom of a bowl. Place half of the vegetables on top of the rice and then top with half of the fish. Sprinkle with sesame seeds. Garnish with avocado, cilantro, and seaweed slivers.

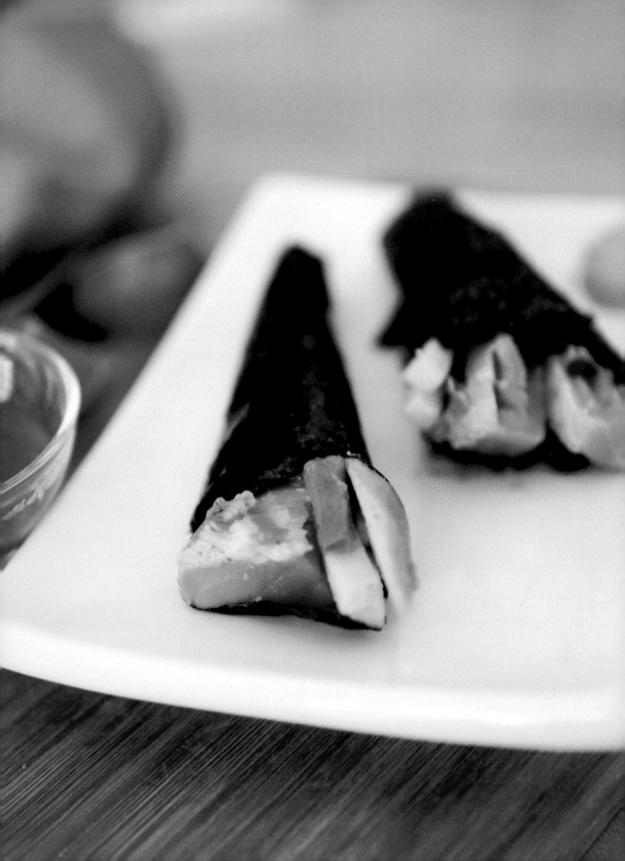

Wild Salmon, Avocado, and Cucumber Hand Rolls (Serves 1)

Keep the night rolling along with the benefits of spicy foods to increase sex drive and fish for heart-healthy fats.

Ingredients

2 tablespoons low-sugar, all-fruit apricot preserves
⅛ teaspoon red pepper flakes or chili paste
2 sheets nori (square seaweed sheets)
½ avocado, sliced thin
½ cup thinly sliced cucumber
4 ounces cooked wild salmon

Directions

- Combine the apricot preserves and red pepper flakes in a small bowl. This will be your dipping sauce.
- Place a nori sheet on a plate or cutting board. Place half of the avocado, cucumber, and wild salmon on half of the nori. Roll up as tightly as possible. Repeat with remaining ingredients. Serve with dipping sauce.

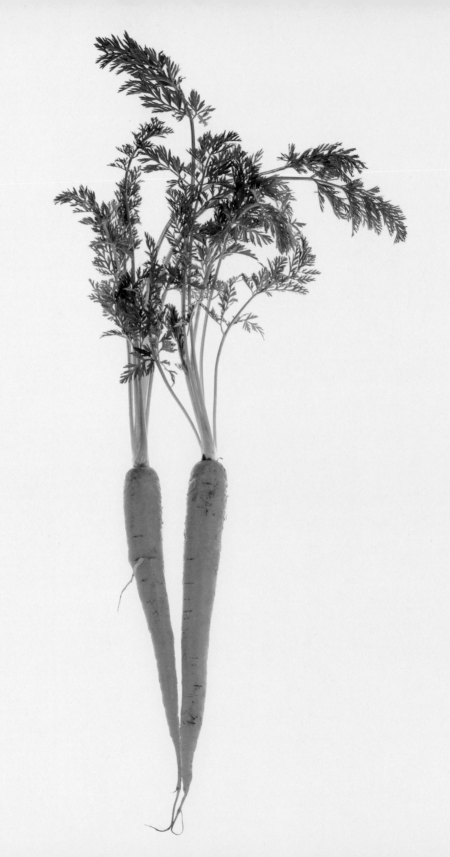

Chapter Eighteen
SEDUCTIVE SIDES

These side dishes are sure to enhance the Exotic Entrees in the previous section, but you can also serve them as a light meal, or between meals.

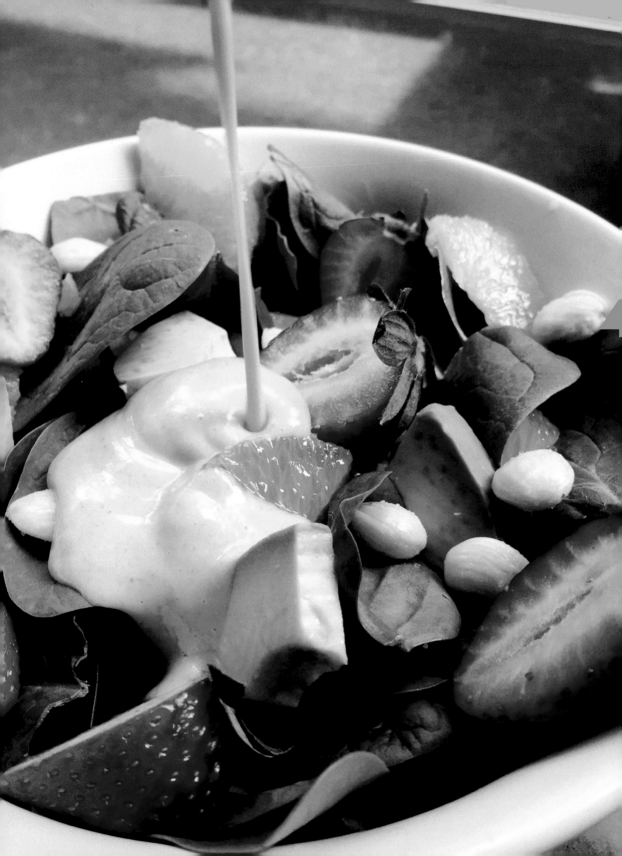

Aphrodisiac Salad with Sexy Fig Dressing *(SERVES 2)*

With lots of healthy fats and spinach for magnesium, this salad is both satisfying and great for sexual health.

Recipe developed by Diana Stobo

Sexy Fig Dressing Ingredients

¼ cup flax seed oil (Diana's choice is Udo's Oil)

¼ cup orange juice, freshly squeezed

2 calimyrna or Kalamata figs, barely covered in water, soaked for 1 hour (save the water!)

1 tablespoon apple cider vinegar

½ teaspoon sea salt

Aphrodisiac Salad Ingredients

1 head butter lettuce, frisee, or organic spinach

1 avocado, diced

1 orange cut into segments

5 organic strawberries, sliced

½ cup Marcona almonds

Directions

- Place all dressing ingredients in high-speed blender and blend for 60 seconds. Add the water from the figs a little at a time to get the desired consistency.
- Place all salad ingredients in large salad bowl and toss with Sexy Fig Dressing.

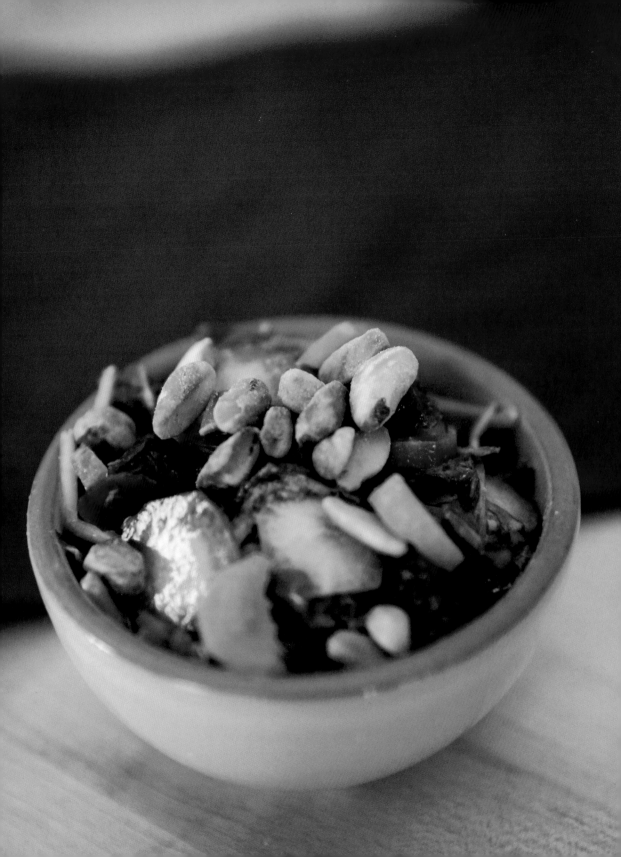

Baby Kale Salad with Roasted Vegetables and Miso-Tahini Dressing (Serves 4)

Make kale part of your regular diet to increase your intake of magnesium to soothe nerves and increase blood flow for those special moments.

Miso-Tahini Dressing Ingredients

1 tablespoon sweet yellow or white miso
1 tablespoon tahini
½ tablespoon low-sodium soy sauce or tamari
1 tablespoon rice vinegar

Baby Kale Salad Ingredients

3 rainbow carrots, peeled and sliced into thin rounds
1 zucchini, sliced into thin rounds
1 tablespoon avocado oil
Pinch of sea salt and pepper
5 ounces baby kale
¼ cup pistachios
¼ cup dried organic cherries, apricots, golden raisins, or dried fruit of choice

Directions

- Combine all dressing ingredients in a mason jar. Place the lid on securely and shake until blended. If a thinner consistency is desired, add more rice vinegar and shake again.
- Heat oven to 375°F. Line a sheet pan with aluminum foil and rub carrots and zucchini with avocado oil. Place carrots and zucchini on the sheet pan and sprinkle with sea salt and pepper. Put the pan in the oven and bake for 15 minutes.
- Place the baby kale in a large mixing bowl. Pour half of the dressing over the salad and massage the dressing into the kale for about 1 minute, or until the kale is tenderized and shrinks in volume.
- Chop roasted vegetables and add to the dressed kale. Add in pistachios and dried fruit.

Note: to make this into a main course, add in grilled chicken or wild salmon.

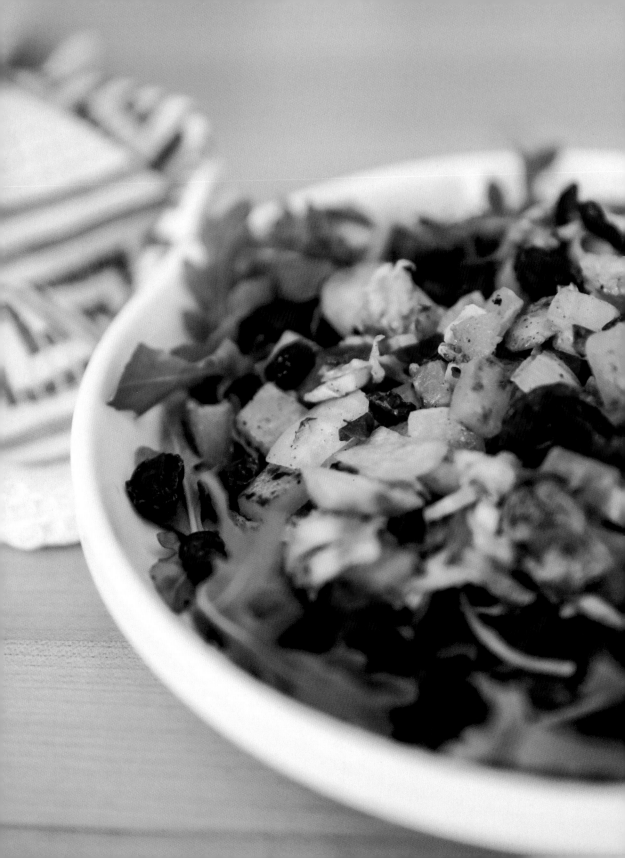

Butternut Squash and Brussels Sprouts Salad with Maple Rosemary Sauce (Serves 4)

The niacin (vitamin B3) in dark, leafy greens helps increase blood flow and the other B vitamins keep you energized throughout the night.

Ingredients

1 tablespoon virgin coconut oil
1 butternut squash, peeled and chopped
½ red onion, chopped
10 Brussels sprouts, sliced thin
Pinch of sea salt and pepper
1 teaspoon chopped rosemary
1 tablespoon maple syrup (Grade A dark amber preferred)
2 tablespoons raw almond butter
1 tablespoon extra-virgin olive oil or avocado oil
2 tablespoons apple cider vinegar
2 cups cooked quinoa
4 cups baby arugula
½ cup pomegranate arils (seeds)

Directions

- Heat a large nonstick skillet over medium-high heat (it is important the heat is not too high) and add coconut oil. When hot, add squash, onion, and Brussels sprouts. Season with sea salt and pepper and cook until veggies are soft, about 7–8 minutes. Remove to a bowl.
- Whisk together rosemary, maple syrup, almond butter, olive oil, and vinegar into a smooth dressing.
- Mix the quinoa, arugula, and pomegranate arils together in a bowl. Place a scoop of cooked quinoa mixture in a bowl and top with veggies and a spoonful of dressing.

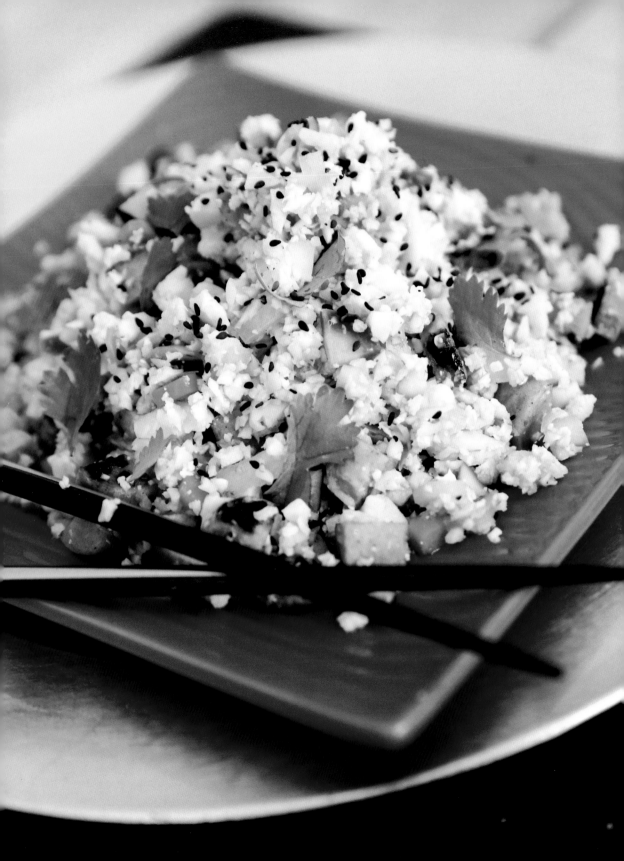

Cauliflower Fried Rice (SERVES 6)

Avocado oil is the concentrated form and has all of the sexual benefits of the whole fruit: energy-boosting B vitamins and healthy fats that give you stamina.

Ingredients

1 head cauliflower, cut into large chunks
1 tablespoon avocado oil
½ sweet yellow onion, chopped
1 each purple, yellow, and orange carrot (if available), peeled and chopped
1 zucchini, chopped
1 large clove garlic, minced
1–2 tablespoons low-sodium tamari or soy sauce
1 teaspoon toasted sesame oil
½ tablespoon rice vinegar
1 green onion, chopped
½ teaspoon black sesame seeds for garnish

Directions

- Place the chunks of cauliflower into the food processor and pulse until very small pieces. Set aside.
- Heat avocado oil in a large nonstick pan. When hot, add the onion, carrots, and zucchini and sauté for 5 minutes. Add garlic and sauté for 1 minute. Add the cauliflower and sauté another 4 minutes. Add the tamari, sesame oil, and rice vinegar and toss to coat. Garnish with green onion and black sesame seeds.

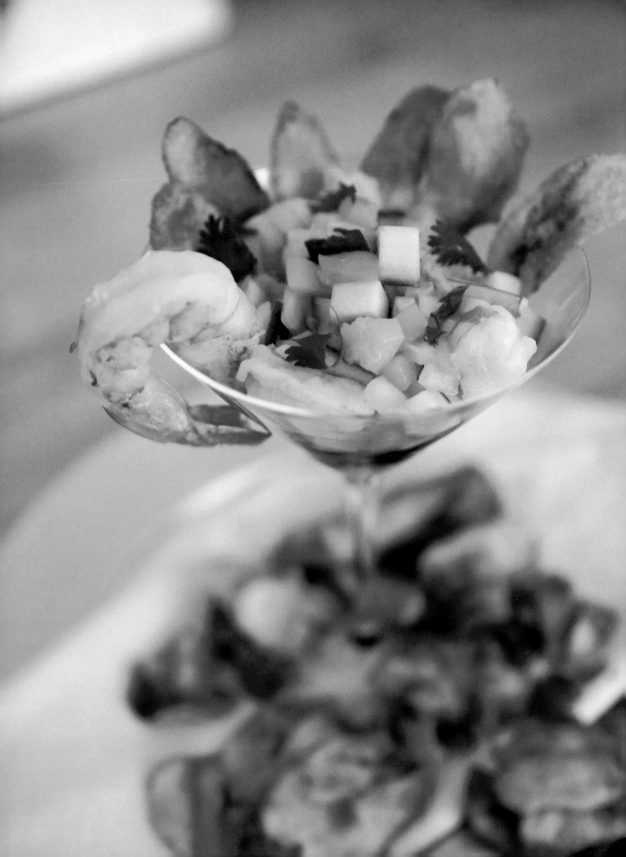

Ceviche with Plantain Chips (SERVES 2)

Onions have been shown to increase sperm count in men and sex drive in both males and females.

Ingredients

8 ounces firm white fish, such as red snapper, rockfish, or shrimp, cleaned

Zest and juice of 1 lemon, 1 lime, and 1 orange

½ sweet yellow onion, diced

½ cup chopped red bell pepper

½ English cucumber, peeled and diced

1 mango, peeled, seeded, and diced

¼ cup chopped cilantro

8–10 store-bought plantain chips

Directions

- Chop the fish into small pieces and place in a glass bowl. Add half the citrus juices and let sit for 20 minutes to "cook" the fish. The acid on raw fish will actually cook the fish without heat.
- Pour off the liquid from the fish and then add the remaining juice, zest, onion, red bell pepper, cucumber, mango, and cilantro. Stir to combine.
- Serve in a bowl or make it fancy and serve in a margarita glass. Garnish with plantain chips.

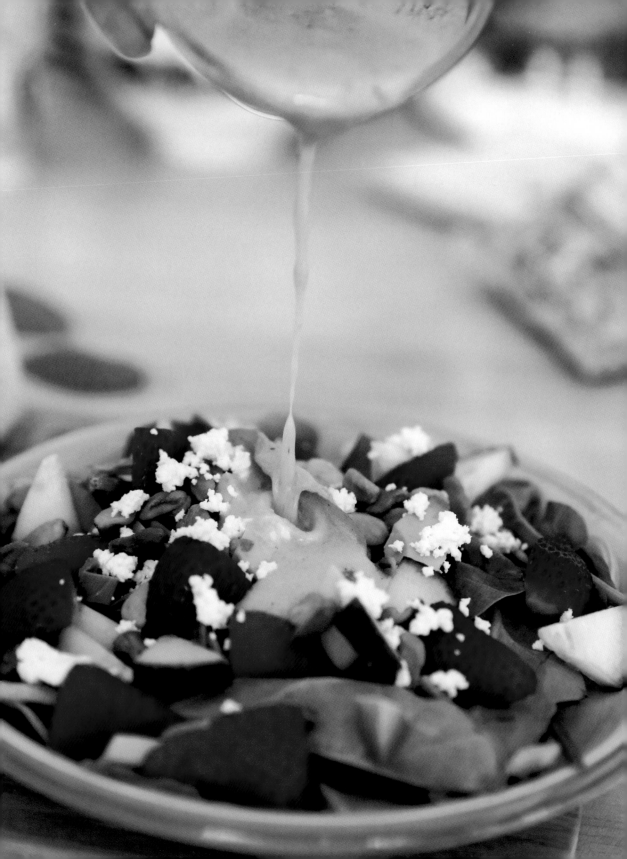

Farmers Market Salad with Lemon Vinaigrette (SERVES 1)

Pistachios act as "erection protection" with the help of the amino acid L-arginine which helps build up nitric oxide, the gas that aids in erection.

Lemon Vinaigrette

Juice and zest of one lemon
1 tablespoon avocado oil
1 teaspoon Dijon mustard
¼ teaspoon cracked lemon pepper

Salad Ingredients

2 cups organic baby spinach
2 basil leaves, chiffonade
4 organic strawberries, chopped
½ medium avocado
¼ cup chopped cucumber
2 tablespoons crumbled goat cheese
2 tablespoons pistachios

Directions

- Place all vinaigrette ingredients in a container with a lid. Shake well until thoroughly mixed.
- Combine baby spinach and basil and toss with half of the dressing.
- Add in strawberries, avocado, cucumber, goat cheese, and pistachios. Add in rest of dressing (if desired) and toss.

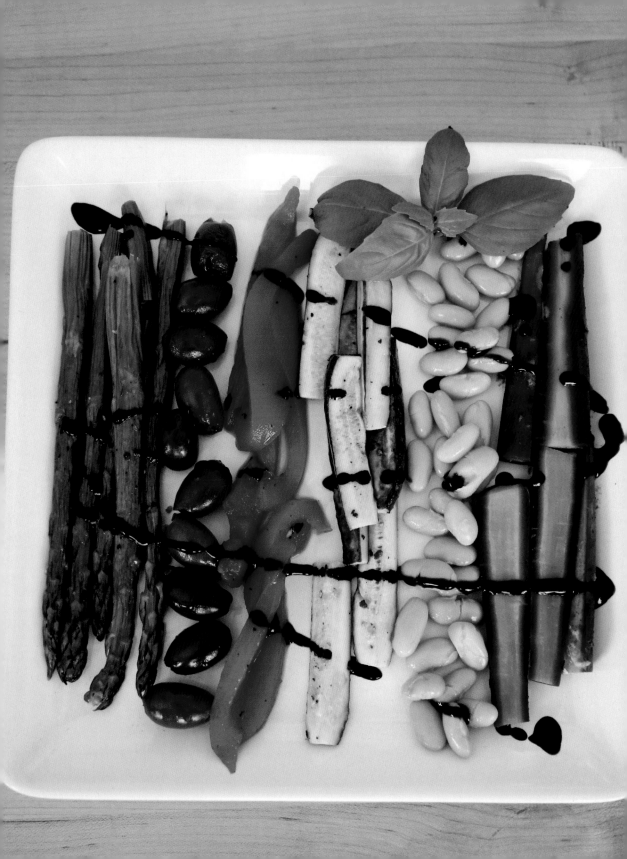

Grilled Vegetable Antipasto Salad with Balsamic Vinaigrette (SERVES 2)

Zucchini, asparagus, cannellini beans, red bell peppers, and parmesan all contain calcium which aids in muscle contraction and firing—an important part of sexual performance.

Ingredients

1 zucchini, sliced
1 red bell pepper
2 carrots (multicolor recommended)
10 asparagus spears
1 tablespoon avocado oil
Sea salt
Lemon pepper
10 Kalamata olives (or substitute your favorite kind)
⅔ cup cannellini beans
4–5 large shavings fresh parmesan off the block
Balsamic glaze
Basil leaves, sliced into ribbons for garnish

Directions

- Heat oven to 375°F. Line a sheet pan with aluminum foil. Place zucchini, pepper, carrots, and asparagus on the sheet pan. Rub with oil and season with 2 pinches each of salt and lemon pepper. Place in the oven and roast for 10 minutes. Remove the asparagus and then roast the remaining vegetables for another 15 minutes.
- Place roasted veggies on a platter in rows and then add the olives and beans. Shave some fresh parmesan cheese on top and drizzle with balsamic glaze and basil leaves.

Note: You may increase or decrease the amount of vegetables based on the number of people you are serving.

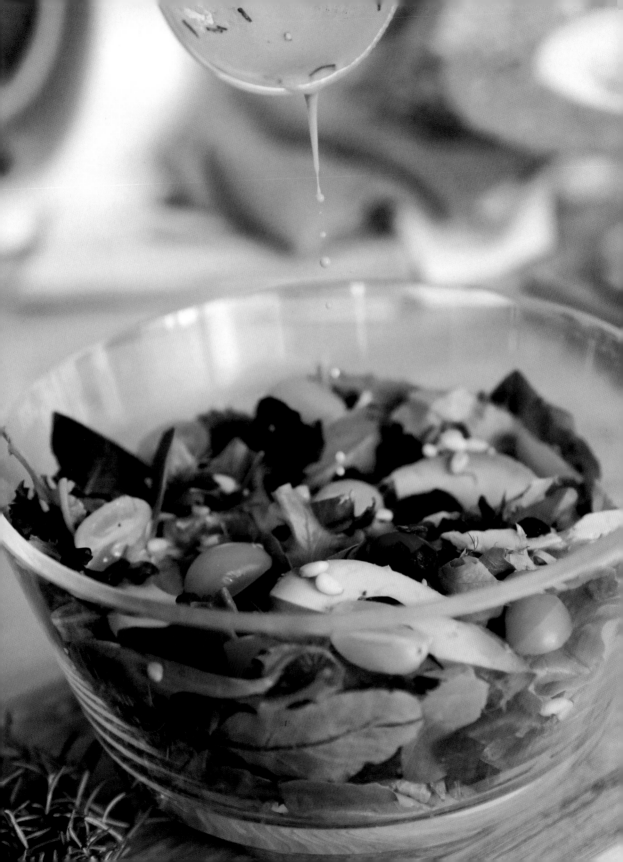

Herbs and Greens Salad   (SERVES 2)

Pine nuts are full of healthy fats and have been shown to improve blood vessel health to keep them efficiently delivering vital nutrients throughout the body.

Dressing Ingredients

2 tablespoons extra-virgin olive oil
    or avocado oil
2 tablespoons red wine vinegar
1 teaspoon Dijon mustard
1 teaspoon minced fresh rosemary
Sea salt and pepper

Spiced Pine Nuts Ingredients

½ teaspoon raw honey
½ teaspoon avocado oil
⅛ teaspoon each smoked paprika,
    cumin, and garlic powder
¼ cup raw pine nuts

Salad Ingredients

2 slices nitrate-free turkey bacon
1 tablespoon fresh rosemary,
    minced
4 cups salad greens
¼ cup dried tart organic cherries
1 cup cherry or grape tomatoes,
    halved
1 large avocado, peeled and sliced

Directions

- Whisk all dressing ingredients together in a mason jar.
- For the pine nuts, combine the honey, oil, and spices in a bowl. Add the raw pine nuts and stir to coat. Heat a small skillet over low heat. When hot, add the pine nuts to the pan and toast for 4 minutes. Remove and set in a bowl to cool down.
- Heat a large skillet over medium heat and cook turkey bacon until done. Remove from pan and chop.
- Place salad greens in a large bowl. Pour ½ of the dressing over greens and toss to coat. Add the bacon, dried cherries, tomatoes, and avocado to the salad. Top with spiced pine nuts.

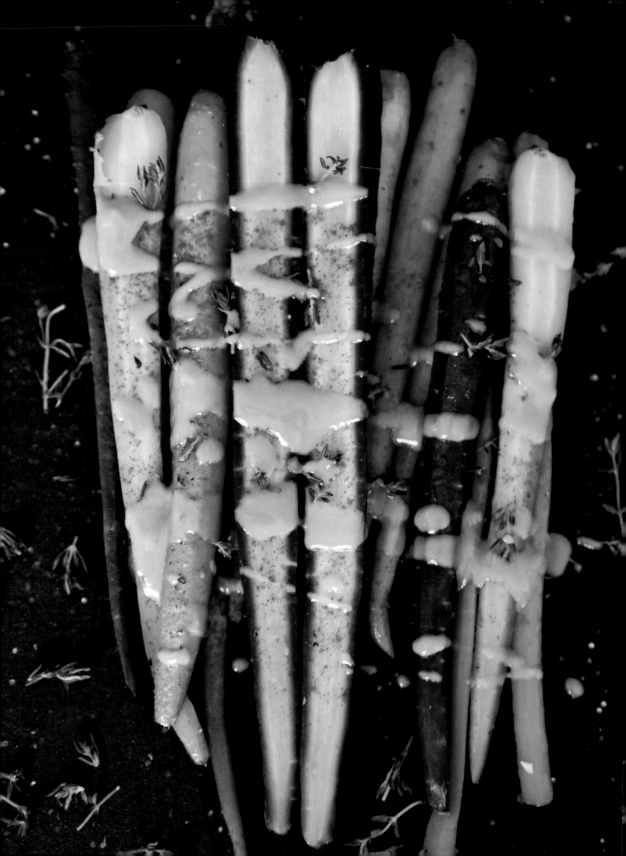

Miso-Maple Glazed Rainbow Carrots (SERVES 4)

Carrots provide a healthy dose of beta-carotene, which is necessary for the synthesis of several sex hormones.

Ingredients

1 tablespoon maple syrup (Grade A dark amber recommended)

1 tablespoon white or yellow miso paste

1 teaspoon toasted sesame oil

1 tablespoon low-sodium tamari or soy sauce

1 tablespoon rice vinegar

½ teaspoon grated ginger

1 bag rainbow carrots, peeled

2 tablespoons chopped mint

Directions

- Combine all but the last two ingredients in a bowl to make your glaze.
- Heat oven to 350°F. Line a baking sheet with aluminum foil and coat with cooking spray.
- Place carrots on the baking sheets and place in oven. Roast for 15 minutes.
- Remove and pour the glaze over the carrots.
- Cook an additional 10–15 minutes or until carrots are soft. Remove and garnish with fresh mint.

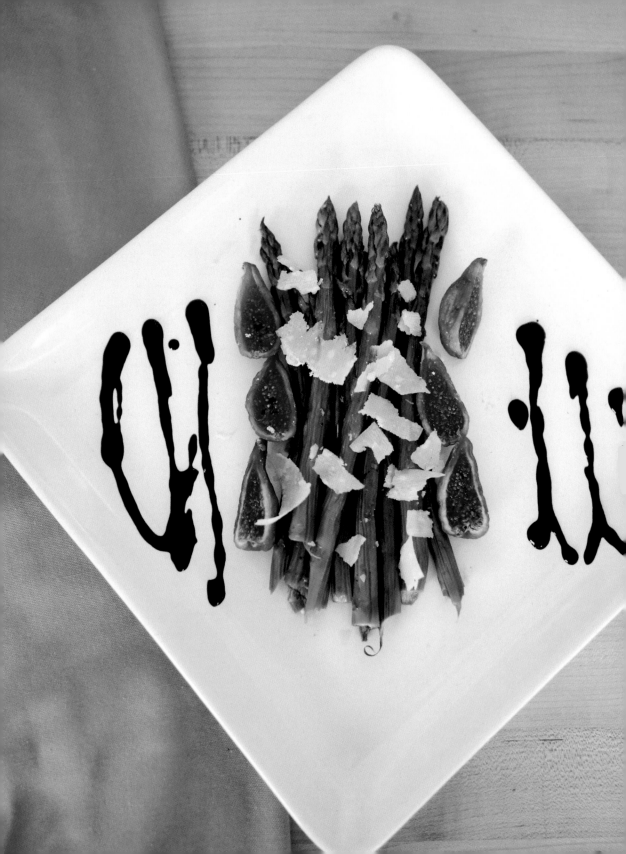

Roasted Asparagus and Figs with Balsamic Glaze (SERVES 4)

Asparagus is rich in vitamin E, also known as the "Sex Vitamin" due to its role in reproductive health.

Ingredients

1 bunch asparagus, with woody ends trimmed off
3–4 fresh figs (or use dried when fresh are not in season)
½ tablespoon avocado oil
¼ teaspoon sea salt
Cracked lemon pepper
Balsamic glaze

Directions

- Heat oven to 350°F. Line a baking sheet with aluminum foil. Toss asparagus and figs with oil and place on the baking sheet. Season with salt and lemon pepper.
- Place in the oven and roast for 10 minutes. Remove and let cool. Transfer to a serving plate and drizzle with balsamic glaze.

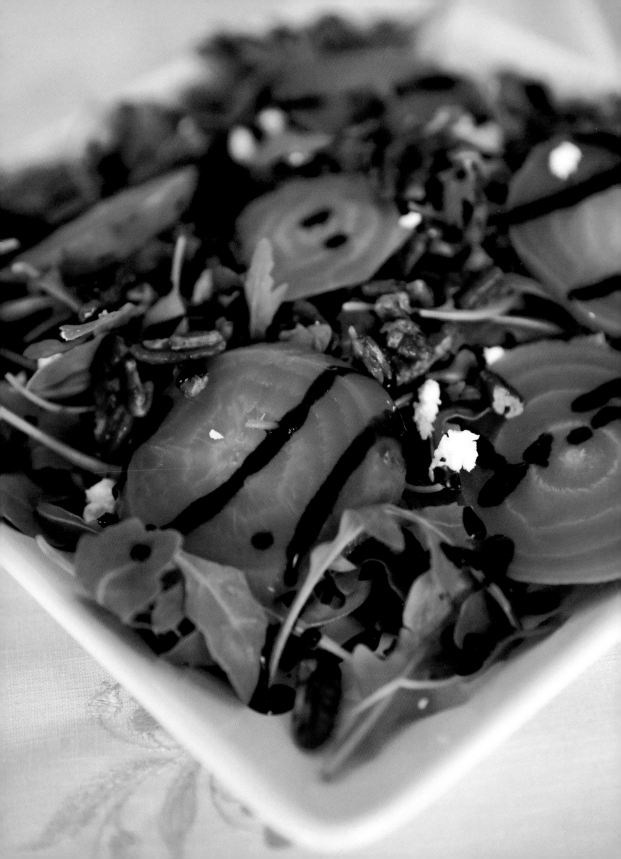

Roasted Beet Salad (SERVES 1)

Cinnamon is a woman's new best friend! This sensual spice has long been used to increase sex drive in women.

Ingredients

2 large organic golden beets
⅛ teaspoon each smoked paprika and cinnamon
Sea salt
1 teaspoon avocado oil
¼ cup raw pecans
3 cups organic baby spinach
½ large avocado, diced
2 tablespoons goat cheese
Balsamic glaze

Directions

- Heat oven to 400°F. Peel the beets and wrap them in aluminum foil. Place in the oven and roast until soft, about 40 minutes. Remove and let cool. Use a paper towel to remove any remaining skin from the beets. Slice into rounds.
- In a mixing bowl add the smoked paprika, cinnamon, sea salt, and avocado oil. Stir and add the pecan pieces. Heat a pan over low heat and add the pecan mixture. Cook 4–5 minutes, shaking the pan as needed to keep from burning.
- Place the baby spinach, beets, avocado, goat cheese, and pecans onto a plate. Drizzle with the balsamic glaze and serve.

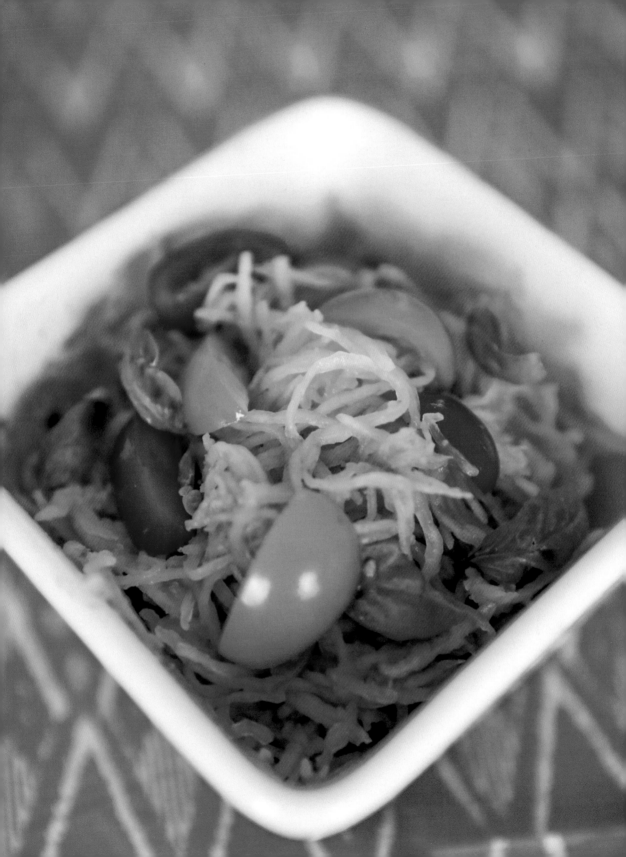

Spaghetti Squash with Tomatoes and Pesto (SERVES 4)

Spaghetti squash packs a super punch of fiber, stabilizing blood sugar, which prevents diabetes and poor circulation.

Ingredients

1 spaghetti squash, halved and seeded
2 cups fresh basil leaves
1 clove garlic
Zest and juice of 1 lemon
2 tablespoons toasted pine nuts
2 tablespoons parmesan cheese
¼ teaspoon cracked lemon pepper
2 tablespoons extra-virgin olive oil
1 cup grape tomatoes
Fresh basil leaves for garnish

Directions

- Heat oven to 375°F. Place squash halves onto a baking sheet, cut side down, and place into oven for 30–45 minutes or until squash is soft when you touch it.
- Place the basil, garlic, lemon zest and juice, pine nuts, parmesan cheese, and lemon pepper into the bowl of a food processor and process until everything is broken down small. With the blender running, slowly add in the olive oil and blend another 30 seconds.
- After the squash comes out of the oven, remove it from the baking sheet to a cutting board to cool for a few minutes. Then, use a fork to scrape the inside of each squash half and you will see the spaghetti strands start to separate. Scoop the strands into a bowl and toss with the pesto. Add the tomatoes to the bowl and top with some fresh basil leaves.

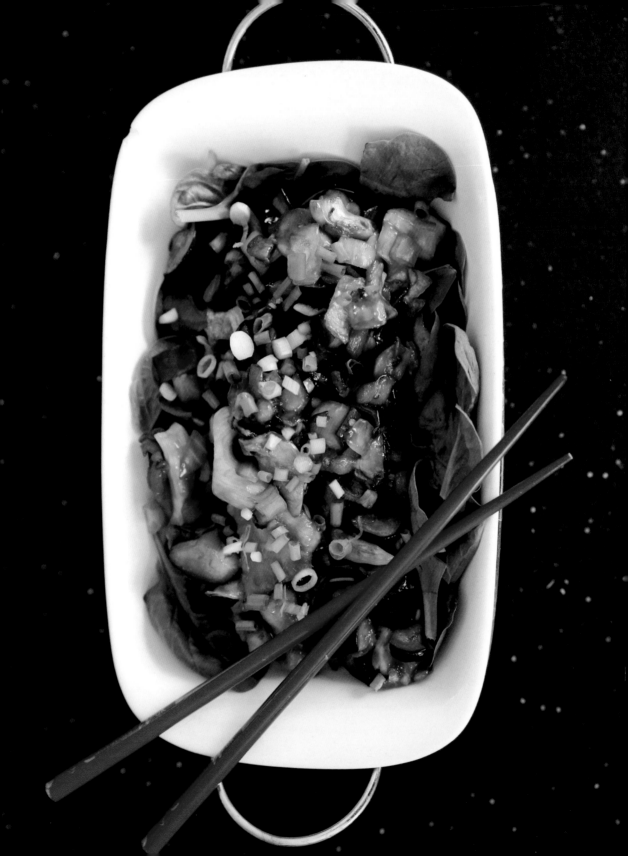

Sticky and Spicy Japanese Eggplant (SERVES 4)

Spice up the night and benefit from the natural vasodilation (widening of blood vessels) which helps blood flow.

Sauce Ingredients

1 teaspoon arrowroot powder
1 tablespoon low-sodium soy sauce or tamari (or coconut aminos sauce)
2 teaspoons Asian sweet chili sauce
1 tablespoon coconut sugar
½ teaspoon toasted sesame oil
¼ teaspoon crushed red pepper

Japanese Eggplant Ingredients

1 tablespoon toasted sesame oil
¼ cup sweet yellow onion, chopped
1 long or 2 short Japanese eggplants, chopped
2 cups sliced oyster or shiitake mushrooms
1–2 cloves minced garlic
½ teaspoon minced ginger
2 green onions, chopped

Directions

- Combine all sauce ingredients in a mason jar. Twist on the lid and shake to combine. Set aside until ready to use.
- Heat the oil in a large non-stick pan over medium-high heat. When hot, add the onion and eggplant. Sauté 4–5 minutes. Add mushrooms, garlic, and ginger, and sauté until eggplant is soft, about 6–7 minutes.
- Shake the sauce, remove the lid, and pour into the skillet. Stir to coat everything. Add the green onions and stir to combine.

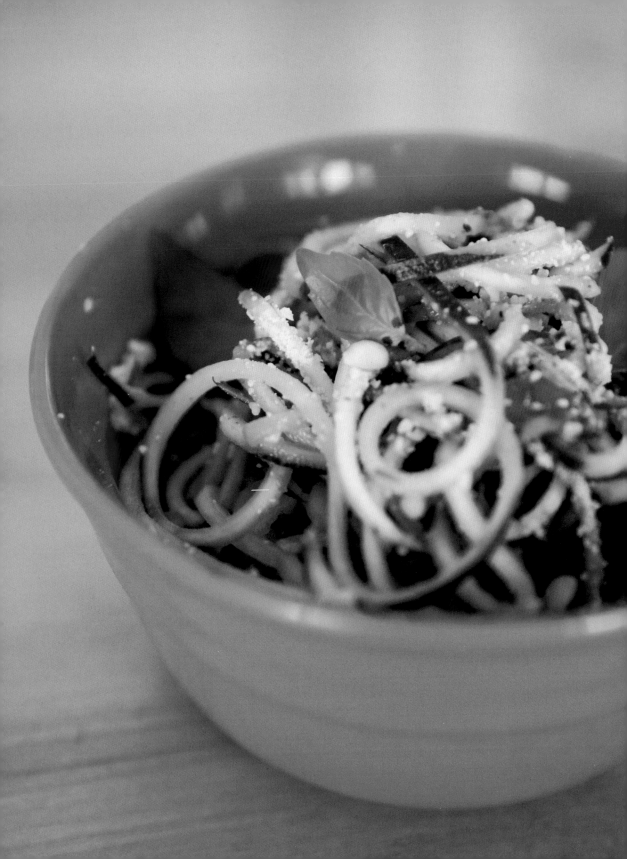

Zucchini Noodles with Basil Pesto (SERVES 2)

Lemons are the ultimate wingman, lending a helping hand with a boost of the antioxidant vitamin C, which combats low sexual stamina in the battlefield of love.

Basil Pesto Ingredients

12 large basil leaves
1 clove garlic, minced
Zest and juice of 1 lemon
2 tablespoons pine nuts
1 tablespoon parmesan cheese
¼ teaspoon cracked lemon pepper
1 tablespoon extra-virgin olive oil

Zucchini Noodles Ingredients

1 tablespoon avocado oil
1 zucchini, spiralized (these are
    also available already packaged,
    if you don't have a spiralizer)
Sea salt
Lemon pepper

Directions

- Add basil leaves, garlic, lemon zest and juice, pine nuts, parmesan cheese, and lemon pepper in a food processor and pulse until chopped. Add olive oil and blend until smooth.
- Add avocado oil to a large pan on high heat. Once hot, add zucchini, sea salt, and lemon pepper.
- Add pesto sauce to zucchini in the pan and toss until well-coated.
- Garnish with pine nuts and serve.

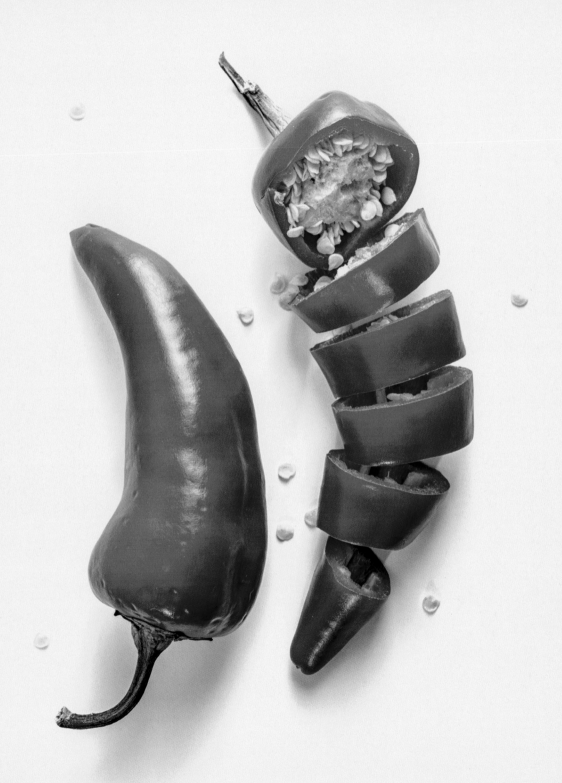

Chapter Nineteen

DOWN AND DIRTY DESSERTS

We all know you may not make it to dessert, but here are some very clean desserts designed to enhance those special moments of connection you love. These make great snacks, too!

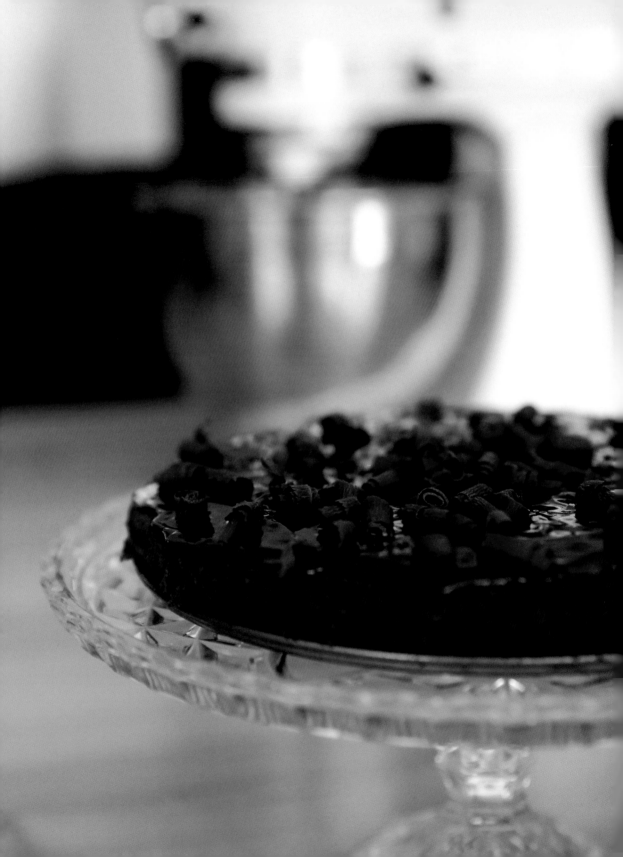

Almond Flour Chocolate Cake (SERVES 8)

Love your honey for years to come by adding almonds into your diet to promote heart health and stabilize blood sugar.

Ingredients

Coconut oil cooking spray
2 large eggs
⅔ cup pure maple syrup (Grade A dark amber)
⅓ cup water
1 tablespoon pure vanilla extract
¼ cup cocoa powder
½ teaspoon salt
2 cups almond flour
½ teaspoon baking soda

Optional Glaze Ingredients

½ cup chopped dark chocolate (with 72% cocoa or more)
1 tablespoon melted coconut oil

Directions

- Heat oven to 350°F. Grease a 9-inch round pan with coconut oil cooking spray.
- In a large bowl, combine eggs, maple syrup, water, and vanilla. Whisk until well incorporated.
- Add the cocoa and salt and mix well. Add the almond flour and baking soda and mix until well combined.
- Pour into baking dish and place in center rack of oven and bake for 25–30 minutes. Remove and let cool.
- For the glaze, place the chopped chocolate in a glass bowl and microwave on high for 30–45 seconds. Stir until smooth, then add the coconut oil and stir until incorporated. Pour over cooled cake and use a spatula to spread evenly.

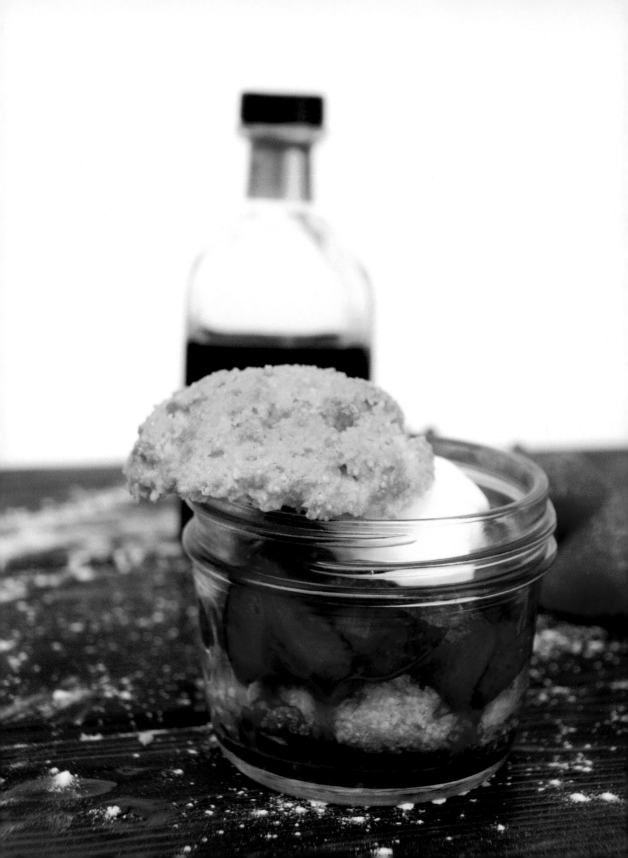

Balsamic Roasted Strawberry Shortcakes (SERVES 12)

Strawberries help support nerve health to keep you feelin' the love.

Ingredients

2 cups fresh organic strawberries, stemmed and halved
2 tablespoons balsamic vinegar
2 tablespoons raw honey
3 eggs
⅓ cup pure maple syrup (Grade A dark amber)
⅓ cup melted virgin coconut oil
1½ teaspoons pure vanilla extract
3½ cups almond flour
¼ teaspoon sea salt
1 teaspoon baking powder
Freshly whipped cream (or vanilla ice cream)

Directions

- Heat oven to 350°F.
- Place the strawberries in a large bowl. Combine the vinegar and honey and pour over berries; toss to coat. Let sit 5 minutes.
- Place berries on a sheet tray lined with parchment paper. Roast 25 minutes. Remove and let cool.
- Combine the eggs, maple syrup, coconut oil, and vanilla extract in a bowl until frothy.
- In another bowl, combine the almond flour, salt, and baking powder. Add the wet ingredients to the dry ingredients and stir to combine to create batter.
- Use a ¼ cup measuring cup to drop batter onto a lined and sprayed baking sheet (or silicone Silpat). Space batter 1 inch apart (they will not spread together). Bake for 25 minutes.
- Cut cakes in half. Remove upper half. On the lower half place some strawberry mixture and 2 tablespoons whipped cream or ice cream. Cover with the upper half.

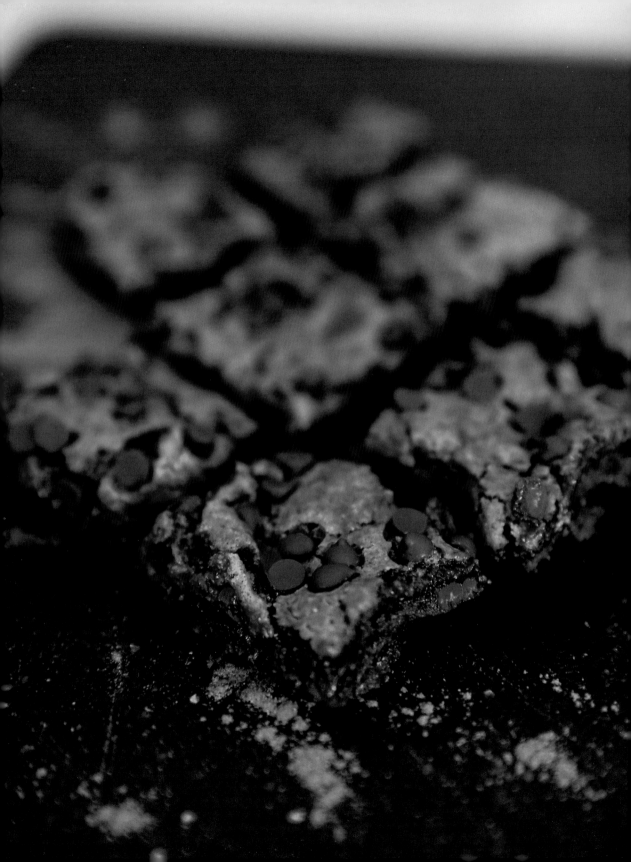

Ooey-Gooey Brownies (Serves 16)

With more antioxidants than green tea or red wine, chocolate and cocoa contain the chemical phenylethylamine, which promotes a sense of well-being and excitement—a bedroom bonus.

Ingredients

Coconut oil cooking spray
1 cup raw smooth cashew butter (may substitute almond or peanut butter)
⅓ cup raw honey
2 tablespoons unsweetened cocoa powder
1 egg
2 tablespoons unsweetened cashew milk (may substitute almond or cow's milk)
1 teaspoon pure vanilla extract
¼ teaspoon cinnamon
Sea salt
1 teaspoon baking powder
2 tablespoons chopped dark chocolate (with 72% cocoa or more)

Directions

- Heat oven to 350°F. Coat an eight-inch square glass baking dish with coconut oil cooking spray.
- Place all of the ingredients, except for the chocolate, in a food processor or use a mixer to blend until smooth. If using a food processor, scrape the resulting batter into a bowl. Fold the chopped chocolate into the batter.
- Pour the batter into the baking dish and bake in the oven for 15 minutes.
- Remove and let cool 15 minutes before slicing.

Chocolate Chip Cookie Dough Bites (Serves 15)

Boost libido with the production of sex hormones after eating the healthy fats from flax seeds.

Ingredients

11 medjool dates, pitted
½ cup raw pecan pieces
1½ tablespoons ground flax seed
Sea salt
¼ teaspoon ground cinnamon
1½ teaspoons pure vanilla extract
3 tablespoons chopped dark
  chocolate (with 72% cocoa or
  more)

Directions

- Place the dates, pecans, flax, salt, cinnamon, and vanilla in the bowl of a food processor. Pulse until well combined (or use a mixer).
- Pour the resulting batter into a bowl. Fold in the chopped chocolate. Roll into bite-sized balls. Enjoy some now and freeze the rest for later.

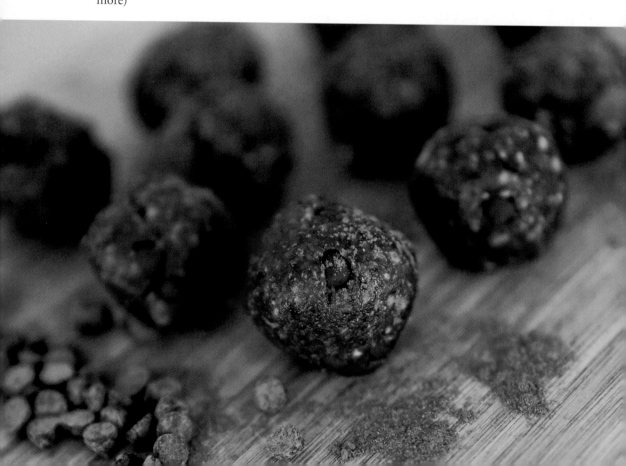

Cinnamon Sautéed Bananas (SERVES 2)

Want to impress your lady with this healthy dessert and get her in the mood? Cinnamon will do just that.

Ingredients

½ tablespoon coconut oil
2 bananas, sliced in half lengthwise
¼ teaspoon cinnamon
Vanilla ice cream or whipped
    coconut cream (optional)

Directions

- Heat the oil in a medium non-stick skillet over medium-high heat.
- When oil is hot, add the bananas, cut side down. Sprinkle with cinnamon. Cook 2–3 minutes or until the bottom is golden.
- Flip and cook an additional 1–2 minutes.
- Place into 2 serving bowls and serve with a scoop of vanilla ice cream or whipped coconut cream.

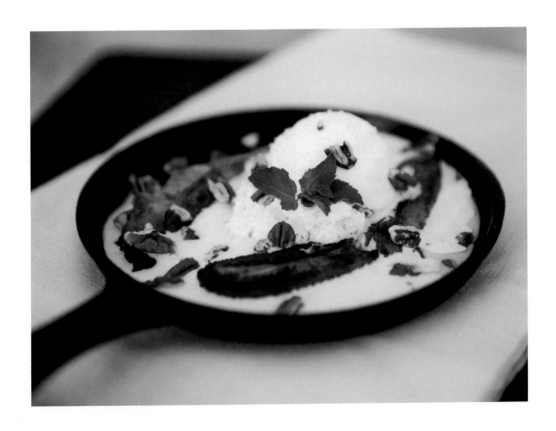

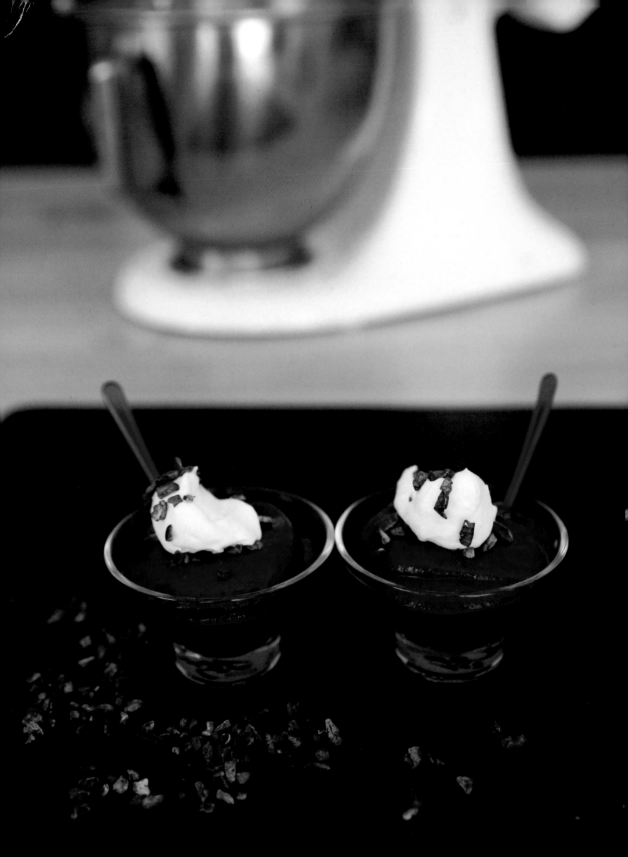

Mexican Chocolate Avocado Mousse (SERVES 4-6)

This chocolate mousse made with avocado and Mexican spice includes healthy fats and is easy, delicious, and dairy free.

Ingredients

2 ripe avocados
½ cup cacao powder or unsweetened cocoa powder
½ cup unsweetened almond milk
¼ cup raw honey, or more to taste
1 teaspoon pure vanilla extract
1 teaspoon cinnamon
¼ teaspoon chili powder (Ancho, a poblano pepper derivative, is preferred)
Sea salt

Directions

- Combine all ingredients in food processor and process until completely smooth. You can also use a mixer.
- Taste and adjust seasonings.
- Spoon into serving dishes and chill to set.

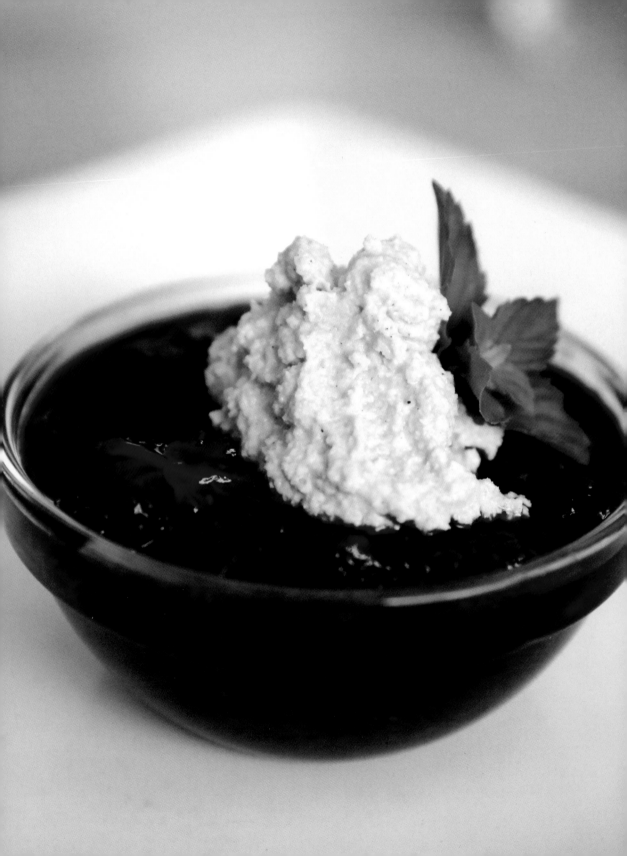

Mixed Berry Bowl with Sweet Cashew Cream (Serves 4)

Small but mighty, chia seeds help decrease inflammation, simultaneously increasing blood flow and circulation.

Ingredients

2 cups frozen organic mixed berries
¾ teaspoon cinnamon, divided
1 tablespoon chia seeds
1 teaspoon pure vanilla extract
1 cup raw cashews, soaked in water at least 4 hours
2 Medjool dates, pitted
Pinch of sea salt
Balsamic glaze (optional)

Directions

- Place frozen berries in a saucepan with ¼ teaspoon cinnamon and bring to a boil. Then reduce to a simmer, cover, and let cook for 10 minutes (the juice will release from the berries as they warm up). Add the chia seeds and another ¼ teaspoon cinnamon, stir in, cover, and let cook another 10 minutes. Stir in the vanilla and remove from the stove to cool and thicken.
- While the berries are cooking, strain the cashews and place in a blender or food processor with the dates and the pinch of sea salt. Pulse to break down the ingredients into a rough paste. Add 1 tablespoon water at a time until a thick cashew cream forms. Add the remaining ¼ teaspoon cinnamon and blend well.
- To assemble the dish, scoop ¼ of the cooked berry mixture into the bottom of each of four bowls. Top with 2 generous tablespoons of cashew cream. If desired, drizzle with balsamic glaze (optional, but highly recommended).

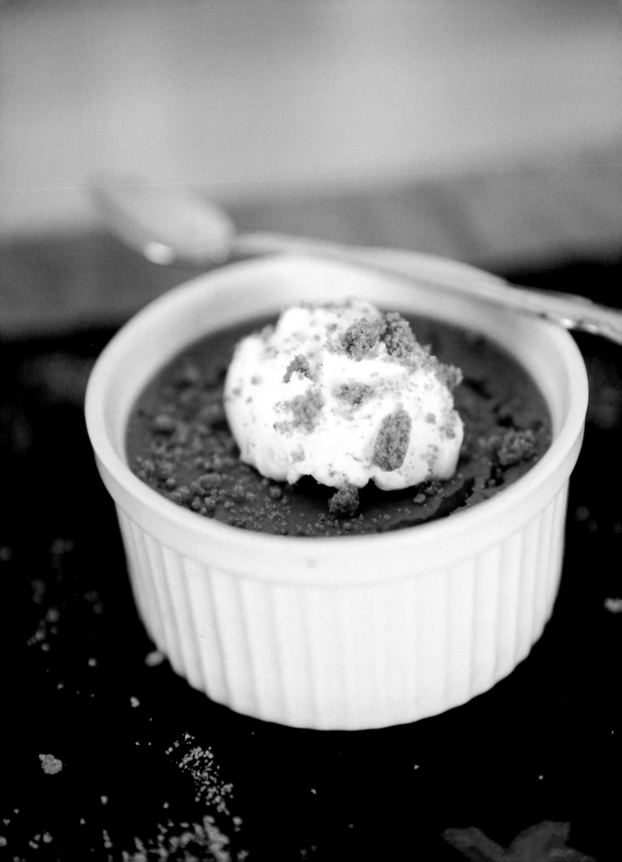

Pumpkin Custard with Coconut Whipped Cream (SERVES 8)

Pumpkin, a robust, testosterone-boosting squash, is high in zinc, which has been linked to increased male sex hormones and improved sperm count.

Pumpkin Custard Ingredients

1 (15 ounce) can pumpkin (not pumpkin pie filling)
12 ounces unsweetened almond milk or coconut milk
1 egg
2 tablespoons coconut sugar
1 teaspoon cinnamon
1 teaspoon pure vanilla extract
Zest of 1 organic orange
½ teaspoon sea salt
1 tablespoon cornstarch or arrowroot powder

Coconut Whipped Cream Ingredients

1 can full-fat coconut milk, refrigerated
1 tablespoon coconut sugar
1 teaspoon pure vanilla extract

Optional Toppings Ingredients

Crushed graham crackers
Pepitas (shelled pumpkin seeds)

Directions

- Heat oven to 350°F. Prepare a 9x13-inch glass baking dish by placing 6–8 ramekins (each holds about ½ cup) inside the baking dish. Heat a tea kettle filled with water or microwave water to a boil. You will need boiling water to create a water bath for this recipe.
- In a large mixing bowl, combine all custard ingredients and whisk until smooth. Pour into the ramekins until they are almost full. Pour the boiling water into the baking dish, surrounding the ramekins. Place the baking dish in oven and bake for 30 minutes.
- While the custard is cooking, make the whipped cream. Open the can of coconut milk and scoop out the hardened milk at the top (transfer any remaining liquid coconut milk out of the can). Place the hardened milk into a mixing bowl and whisk until smooth and starting to thicken. Add the sugar and vanilla and whip another minute. Set aside in the refrigerator to keep cold.
- Remove the cooked custard carefully from the oven and set on the counter or stove top. Make sure to use an oven mitt or oven glove to remove the ramekins from the hot water. Let cool 10–15 minutes.
- Serve with a dollop of coconut whipped cream, some crushed graham crackers, and a few pepitas.

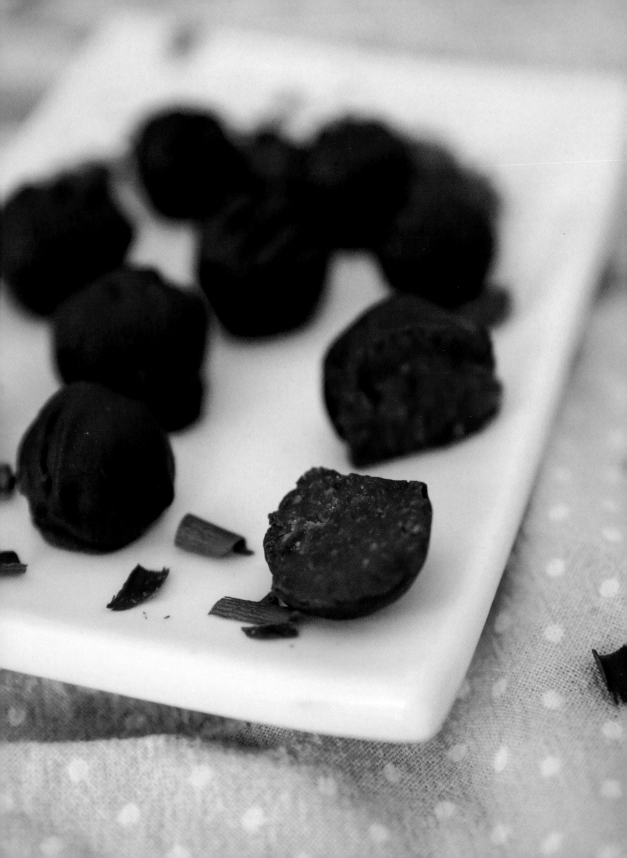

Sweet and Spicy Chocolate Truffles (Serves 15)

Not only are dates a good natural sweetener that avoids blood sugar spikes and prevents circulation problems, but they are also rich in iron, which helps regulate ovulation in women.

Ingredients

14 Medjool dates, pits removed
2 tablespoons raw almond butter
1 teaspoon pure vanilla extract
¼ teaspoon cinnamon
⅛ teaspoon ancho chili powder
Sea salt
1 cup chopped dark chocolate (with 70 percent cocoa, or more)

Directions

- Add dates and almond butter to your food processor. Pulse 20 times or until dates are chopped. Add the vanilla, cinnamon, chili powder, and salt, and pulse another 10 times. You want the mixture to be well-blended and a little bit smooth.
- Prepare a piece of wax paper on a large plate. Use a tablespoon to measure out portions and roll them in your hands to form a ball. Set aside.
- Put the chopped chocolate in a glass bowl and microwave 1 minute. Remove and stir until smooth.
- Dip one date ball at a time in the melted chocolate and lift out with a fork or slotted spoon. Allow the excess chocolate drip back into the bowl. Place the truffle onto the wax paper-lined plate. Repeat with remaining balls.
- Let truffles harden in the freezer for 15 minutes.
- Store in a zip top bag in the refrigerator and enjoy all week (if they last that long).

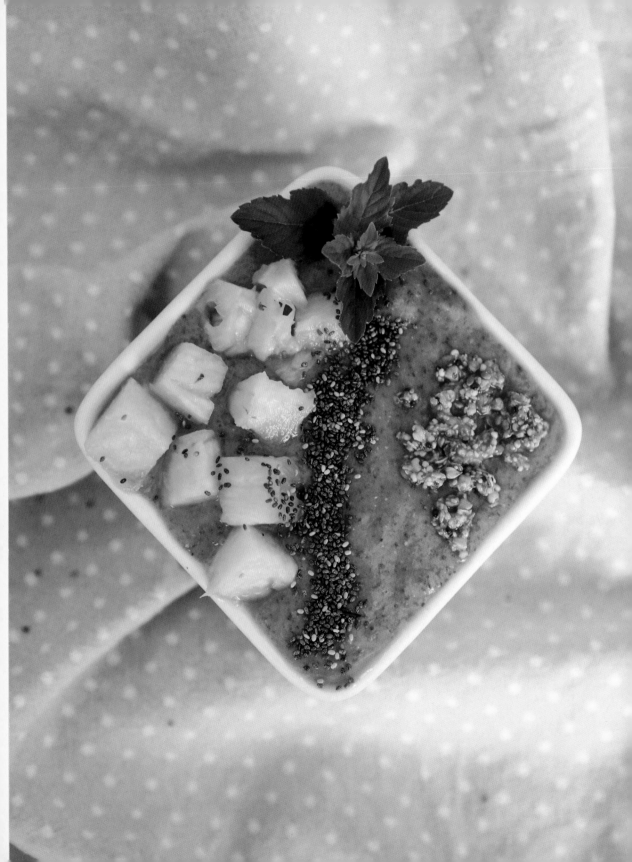

Berry Avocado Smoothie Bowl (Serves 2)

Oats provide healthy fiber and help blood flow. Avocado provides healthy fat and strawberries add flavonoids, both of which support male and female sexual health.

Smoothie Ingredients

1 cup frozen organic strawberries
1 cup pineapple chunks
1 avocado, pitted
⅔ cup almond milk
2 tablespoons chia seeds

Crumble Topping Ingredients

2 tablespoons raw oats
2 teaspoons chia seeds
2 teaspoons hemp seeds
2 teaspoons millet
1 tablespoon raw honey

Directions

- Place all smoothie ingredients into a blender and cover. Blend on high until smooth.
- In a separate bowl, mix crumble topping ingredients until sticky and crumbly. Garnish on top of smoothie bowls.

Blueberry Pie Smoothie (SERVES 2)

Blueberries are another natural Viagra® and great for overall health.

Recipe developed by Tess Masters, The Blender Girl

Ingredients

2 cups unsweetened almond milk
½ cup raw unsalted cashews
¼ cup rolled oats
¼ cup chopped pitted dates, plus
    more to taste
1 tablespoon chia seeds
1 teaspoon pure vanilla extract
1 teaspoon fresh lemon juice
½ teaspoon ground cinnamon
2 cups frozen organic blueberries

Directions

- Throw everything into your blender in the order listed, and blast on high for 30 to 60 seconds until smooth and creamy.

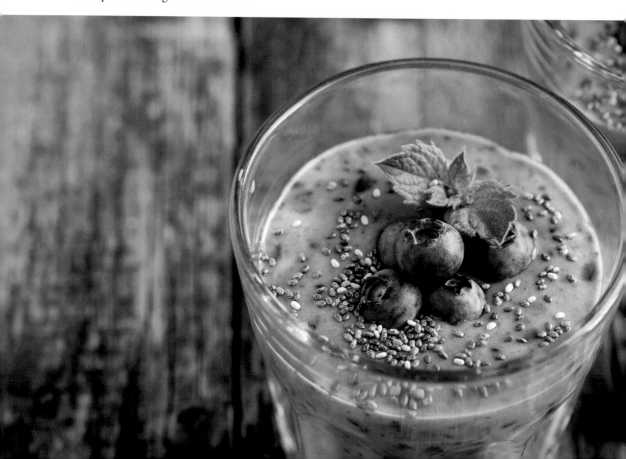

Blueberry Smoothie (SERVES 2)

Want to live a medication-free life? Add blueberries to your diet to get the same benefits as the little blue pill (Viagra®).

Ingredients

1 cup unsweetened almond milk
½ cup frozen organic blueberries
½ frozen banana
Zest of 1 lemon
1 tablespoon lemon juice
1 tablespoon chia seeds

Directions

- Place all ingredients into a blender and blend on high until smooth.

  Optional: add a scoop of your favorite protein powder.

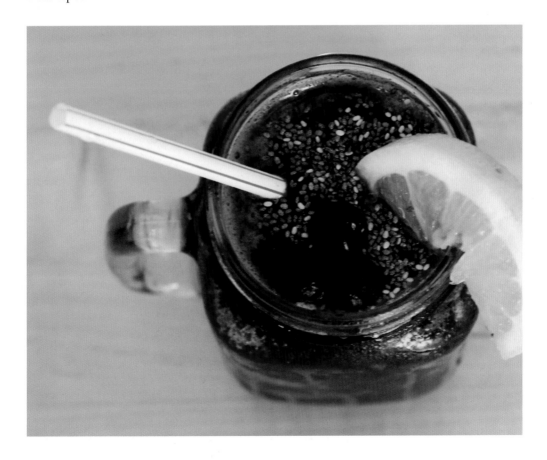

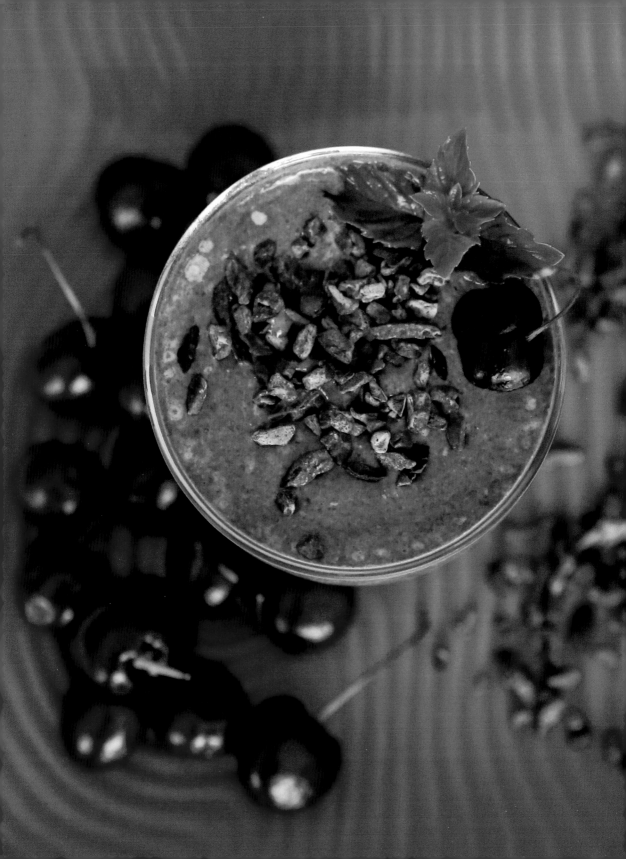

Chocolate Cherry Smoothie (SERVES 1)

Avoid the sugar crash of all-fruit smoothies by adding in lean protein powder, to keep you mentally sharp and physically ready for action.

Ingredients

1 cup unsweetened almond milk
1 cup frozen organic cherries
1 scoop collagen protein powder
   (grass-fed)
1 tablespoon unsweetened cocoa
   powder
1 tablespoon chia seeds
1 drop sweetener (Stevia® is a good
   choice)

Directions

• Place all ingredients into a blender and blend until smooth.

Chocolate, Peanut Butter, Banana Smoothie (Serves 1)

With natural fat from nuts, feel-good dopamine-producing chocolate, potassium from the banana, and protein, this smoothie is high on the list for sexual health.

Ingredients

½ cup unsweetened almond milk

1 scoop chocolate whey protein powder

2 tablespoons peanut butter (can substitute almond or cashew butter)

1 frozen banana

1 tablespoon cacao nibs

Directions

- Combine the milk, protein powder, peanut butter, and banana in a blender and blend until smooth and thick. If it's too thin, add some crushed ice and blend again.
- Pour into a bowl and top with cacao nibs.

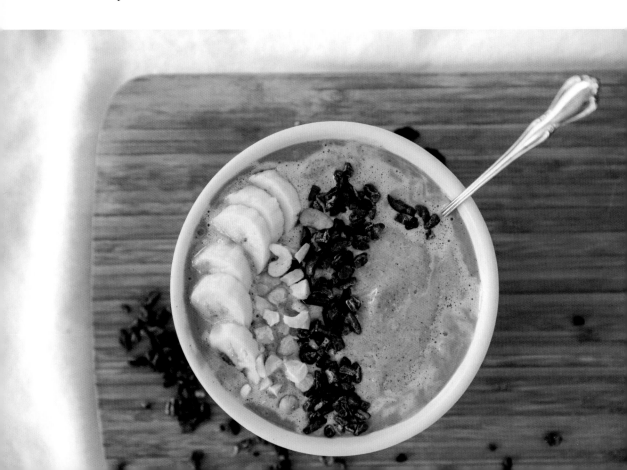

Creamsicle Bliss Dairy-Free Milkshake with Maca (SERVES 2)

Diana Stobo explained that maca is renowned for its hormone-balancing and libido-enhancing properties. It also helps produce stamina in athletes, a real plus in the bedroom.

Recipe developed by Diana Stobo

Ingredients
- 1 cup vanilla coconut-milk ice cream (find it at most health food stores)
- 1½ cups freshly squeezed orange juice
- ½ teaspoon maca powder
- Dash of vanilla powder

Directions
- Blend all ingredients in high-speed blender for 60 seconds.

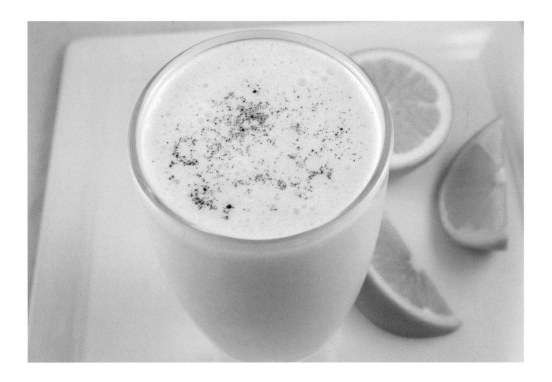

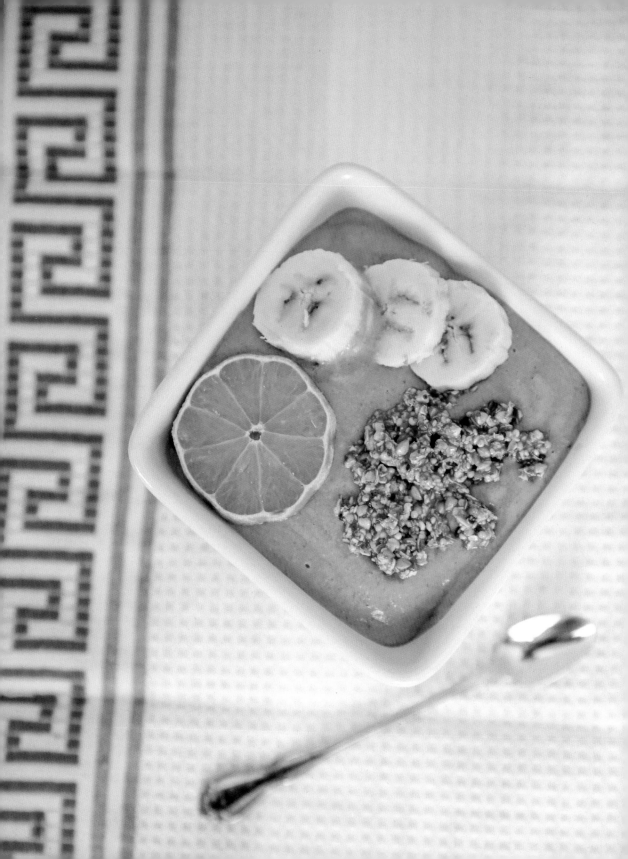

Key Lime Pie Smoothie Bowl with Crumble Topping (SERVES 2)

Avoid the libido-killing, heart-damaging trans fats found in high amounts in pie crust by making this heart-healthy alternative.

Ingredients

2 frozen bananas
½ cup raw cashews
½ cup organic spinach
2 tablespoons unflavored protein powder
3 teaspoon flaxseed meal
¾ teaspoon pure vanilla extract
Juice of 4 limes
Zest of 2 limes
Crumble topping from page 169

Directions

- Place frozen bananas, raw cashews, spinach, protein powder, flaxseed, vanilla, and lime juice in a blender. Add a bit of the lime zest, setting aside some to use as topping.
- Place the lid on the blender and blend on high until smooth. Pour into two bowls and let set in the refrigerator for 25 minutes to thicken.
- In a separate bowl, mix crumble topping ingredients until sticky and crumbly.
- Place crumble and remaining lime zest on top of smoothie bowls and enjoy!

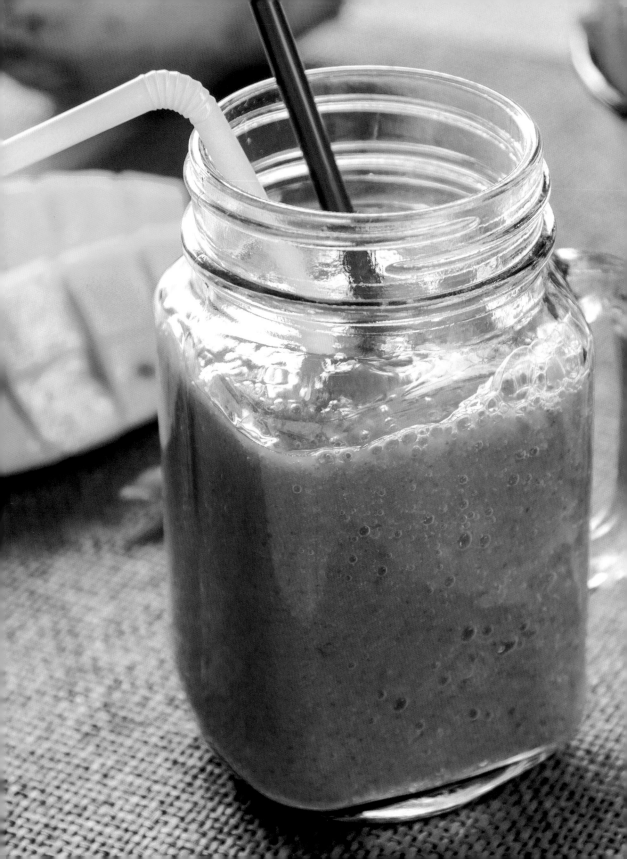

Mango Magic (SERVES 2)

This is an easy and tasty way to get spinach, which contains arginine. Arginine is an amino acid that converts in your system to nitric oxide, which helps guys initiate and maintain erections and aids blood flow to a woman's vaginal area.

Recipe developed by Tess Masters, The Blender Girl

Ingredients

1½ cups raw coconut water or filtered water

1 cup organic baby spinach

½ cup cilantro leaves

2 tablespoons chopped cucumber

2 teaspoons finely chopped red onion

1 teaspoon finely chopped jalapeño pepper, plus more to taste

¼ teaspoon finely grated lime zest, plus more to taste

2 tablespoons fresh lime juice, plus more to taste

¼ teaspoon sea salt, or more to taste

3 cups frozen mango

5 drops alcohol-free liquid sweetener (like stevia), or more to taste (optional)

Directions

- Throw everything into your blender in the order listed, and blast on high for 30 to 60 seconds until smooth.

Mango, Lemon, Turmeric Smoothie (Serves 2)

Turmeric is a powerhouse of antioxidants (apparent by its color) which helps improve prostate health in men.

Ingredients

1½ cups frozen mango
¾ cup almond milk
½ cup kefir
⅓ cup carrots
¼ avocado
⅛ teaspoon turmeric
Juice and zest from 1 lemon

Directions

- Add all ingredients to a blender and blend on high until smooth.

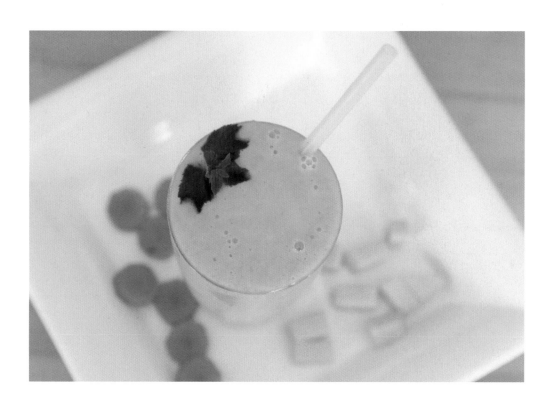

Pink Pleasure (SERVES 2)

With apples and beets, both sexual health boosters, this smoothie is an easy way to share the love.

Recipe developed by Tess Masters, The Blender Girl

Ingredients

1 cup raw coconut water or
   filtered water
1 organic apple, skin on, cored
   and chopped
1 medium raw red beet, peeled
   and chopped (steamed if using
   a conventional blender)
½ small avocado
¼ teaspoon grated lemon zest
2 tablespoons fresh lemon juice
1 teaspoon minced fresh ginger,
   plus more to taste
2 cups frozen pineapple

Directions

- Throw everything into your blender in the order listed, and blast on high for 30 to 60 seconds until smooth.

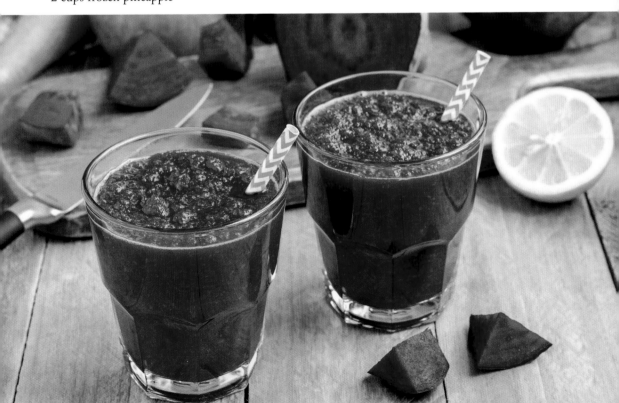

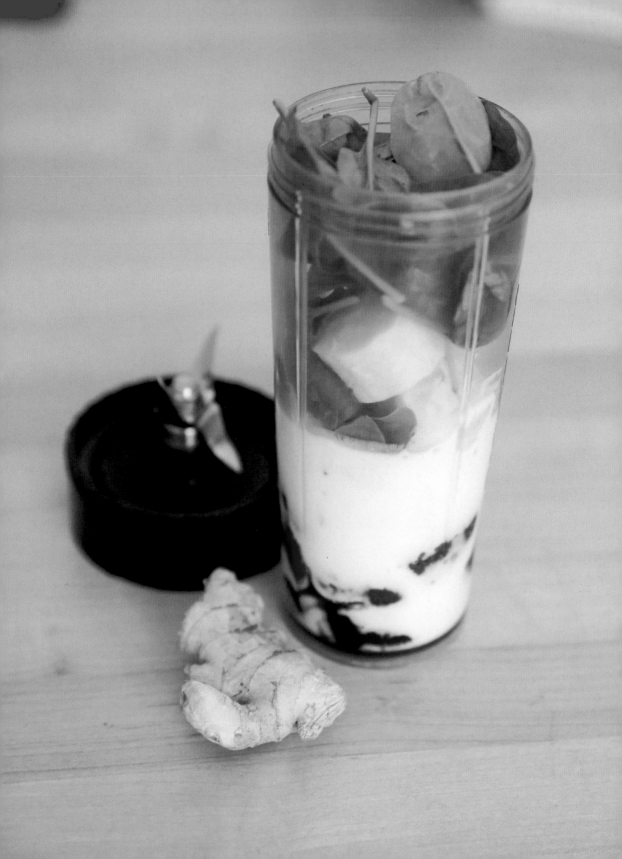

Raspberry and Greens Smoothie with Ginger (Serves 1)

This is a great way to get ginger, with its antioxidant and anti-inflammatory benefits.

Ingredients

1 frozen banana
¾ cup frozen raspberries
⅔ cup kefir
½ cup organic spinach
½ teaspoon vanilla extract
⅛ teaspoon fresh, grated ginger

Directions

- Place all ingredients into a blender and place the lid on. Blend on high until smooth.

Red Romp (SERVES 2)

Watermelon, nature's Viagra®, is the delicious basis for this smoothie.

Recipe developed by Tess Masters, The Blender Girl

Ingredients

3½ cups chopped seedless watermelon

½ medium organic red bell pepper, seeded

Pinch of cayenne pepper, plus more to taste

2 cups frozen organic strawberries

Directions

- Throw everything into your blender in the order listed, and blast on high for 30 to 60 seconds until smooth.

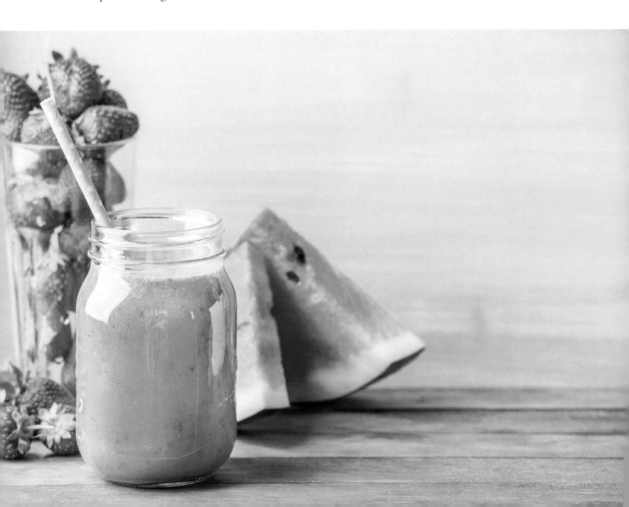

Vanilla Dairy-Free Milkshake with Maca (SERVES 2)

Diana Stobo, explained that maca is renowned for its hormone-balancing and libido-enhancing properties. It also helps produce stamina in athletes, a real plus in the bedroom.

Recipe developed by Diana Stobo

Ingredients

1½ cups vanilla coconut-milk ice cream (found at most health food stores)

1 cup almond milk (or your favorite nut or seed milk)

2 medjool dates, pitted

1½ teaspoons maca powder

1 teaspoon vanilla powder

Directions

- Blend all ingredients in a high-speed blender until smooth and creamy.

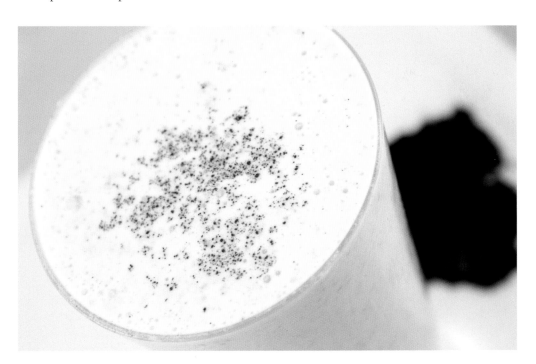

Part Seven

RESOURCES

This book was a whirlwind tour of clean eating, dirty sex, and feelings of gratitude to all who shared their time and talent to create this health resource for you. To assist your continued learning, all the experts featured in this book, along with some products and organizations, are included here. Please visit the websites provided to learn more about topics of interest. To hear great interviews with these experts, and many others, go to my website www.itsyourhealthwithlisadavis.com. Speaking of continued learning, be sure to check out the *Clean Eating, Dirty Sex* podcast and *The Clean Eating, Dirty Sex Total Makeover* offered by Erin and me by going to www.cleaneatingdirtysex .com.

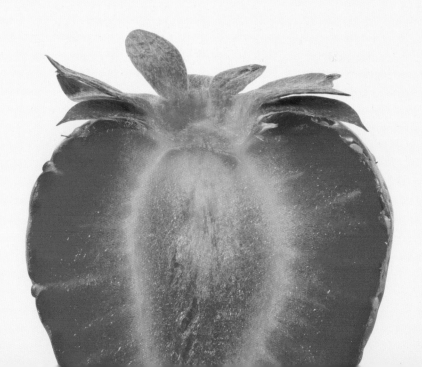

RENOWNED HEALTH EXPERTS

Words cannot adequately express my gratitude to the following individuals. They not only contributed to this book, but their work in the world increases the health and happiness of so many people on the planet. Thank you, thank you, thank you!

Anami, Kim

www.KimAnami.com

Kim Anami is a sex and relationship coach and a vaginal weight lifter. She teaches women how to tone their vaginas and strengthen themselves for great sex. Her coaching is a spiritual synthesis of two decades of Tantra, Taoism, Osho, transpersonal psychology, philosophy, and a host of quantum growth-accelerating practices she uses to propel clients into higher stratospheres of connection, intimacy, energy and creativity. Her VIP intensives have become the stuff of legends, within an elite coterie of society. Her musings on love, life, and sex have graced *Playboy*, *Elle*, *Oprah Magazine*, *Marie Claire*, *Allure*, *Glamour*, *Women's Health*, *Shape*, *Cosmopolitan*, *Self*, *Flare*, *The Sunday Times* (UK), *The Daily Mirror* (UK), *The Daily Mail* (UK), *The Daily Express* (UK), *The Independent* (UK), *GQ*, *FHM*, *Maxim*, *Metro*, *In Touch*, *People*, *Closer*, *Grazia*, *The Huffington Post*, *The Huffington Post Live*, *Salon*, *Yahoo*, *BuzzFeed*, *Mashable*, national talk shows from E! Network and CNN to NPR, and various international radio and television programs around the globe.

Asprey, Dave

https://blog.bulletproof.com

Dave Asprey is a Silicon Valley investor and technology entrepreneur who spent two decades and over $1 million to hack his own biology. Dave lost one hundred pounds without counting calories or excessive exercise, used techniques to upgrade his brain and lift his IQ by twenty points, and lowered his biological age while learning to sleep more efficiently in less time. Learning to do these seemingly impossible things transformed him into a better entrepreneur, a better husband, and a better father. Dave is the creator of the widely popular *Bulletproof Coffee*, host of the #1 health podcast *Bulletproof Radio*, and author of the *New York Times* bestselling books *The Bulletproof Diet* and *Head Strong*. Through his work Dave provides information, techniques, and keys to taking control of and improving your biochemistry, your body, and your mind so they work in unison, helping you execute at levels far beyond what you'd expect, without burning out, getting sick, or allowing stress to control your decisions.

Bond, Ward

www.drwardbond.com

Ward Bond, PhD, is widely known from his writings, television and radio hosting, appearances, and lectures as one of America's most prominent authorities on the use of natural health cures to combat problems of our health and to head off potential problems associated with aging.

Dr. Bond has been hosting the daily television program *Dr. Bond's Think Natural* for the last twelve years, which airs across the United States in 46 million households on CTN, DirecTV (Channel 376), and Dish TV (Channel 267). Dr. Bond has currently filmed over 2,000 episodes of *Think Natural*. Dr. Bond has appeared on many ABC, NBC and Fox affiliates, and DayStar's Celebration, discussing the benefits of natural health.

Botros, Nathalie

www.thebon-vivantgirl.com
Nathalie Botros is a certified health coach and psychotherapist who was born in Lebanon, raised in Turkey, and educated in Switzerland. She played and worked in Italy before eventually landing in New York City, where she lives today. She has never been a skinny girl, but it wasn't until she moved to NYC that she experienced the biggest weight gain of her life. It was time to fuse her health coach training with her psychotherapist mind to blow up the pattern of binge and purge. Nathalie is the author of *If You Are What You Eat, Should I Eat a Skinny Girl?* Her brand is the *Bon Vivant Girl*.

Boz, Wesley

www.MusicAndDance.com
www.CarolinaDanceClub.com
Wesley Boz is an award-winning swing dancer and DJ, and co-owns Music and Dance Productions and Carolina Dance Club with his wife, Debbie Ramsey.

Britton, Patti

www.SexCoachU.com
Patti Britton, PhD, MPH, FAACS, ABS, ACS, ACSE, is a national board-certified clinical sexologist and is co-founder of Sex Coach University, a credentialing and training institute on sex coaching. She is author of *The Art of Sex Coaching: Expanding Your Practice.*

Breus, Michael

www.thesleepdoctor.com
Michael J. Breus, PhD, America's Sleep Doctor™, is a clinical psychologist and both a Diplomate of the American Board of Sleep Medicine and a Fellow of the American Academy of Sleep Medicine. At age thirty-one, he was one of the youngest people to have passed the board and, with a specialty in sleep disorders, is one of only 168 psychologists in the world with his credentials and distinction. Dr. Breus is on the clinical advisory board of *The Dr. Oz Show* and appears regularly on the show.

Burch, Candace

www.yourhormonebalance.com
Candace is a hormone health educator whose mission is to educate and empower women to direct their own path to hormone balance. Candace uses saliva test results as a guide to natural hormone relief and rebalancing. In consultations, Candace covers everything from lifestyle

improvements in diet, sleep, exercise, and stress control to the judicious use of high quality over-the-counter support supplements, herbs, and/or bioidentical hormones as needed.

Cantkier, Lisa

www.healthfulcommunications.com
Lisa Cantkier, CHN, is a nutritionist, nutrition educator, and nutrition/health writer. She enjoys writing about the latest health research findings. Living with the challenges of celiac disease for a lifetime has taught Lisa that every bite matters—food is one of the most important aspects of health and it can either harm or help us. Lisa is also the coauthor of *The Paleo Diabetes Diet Solution* (with Jill Hillhouse), a cookbook that aims to help prevent and manage Type 2 diabetes and blood sugar problems. It includes 125 delicious and wholesome recipes that are all free of gluten, grains, sugar, and dairy.

Cates, Trevor Holly

www.TheSpaDr.com
Dr. Trevor Cates is a nationally recognized naturopathic doctor, also known as The Spa Dr. She was the first woman licensed as a naturopathic doctor in the state of California and was appointed by former governor Arnold Schwarzenegger to California's Bureau of Naturopathic Medicine Advisory Council. She has worked with world-renowned spas, and sees patients in her private practice in Park City, Utah, with a focus on graceful aging and glowing skin. She has been featured on *The Doctors*, *Extra*, *First for Women*, and *Mind Body Green*, and is host of *The Spa Dr.* iTunes podcast. Dr. Cates believes the key to healthy skin is inner and outer nourishment with non-toxic ingredients. She is the author of *Clean Skin from Within*: *The Spa Doctor's Two-Week Program to Glowing, Naturally Youthful Skin*. Dr. Cates' The Spa Dr. skin care and supplement lines are formulated with natural and organic ingredients designed to help you achieve the clean and natural path to confidence and beautiful skin.

Ciminelli, Susan

www.SusanCiminelli.com
Susan Ciminelli is a holistic health, beauty, and wellness guru with thirty-five years experience. Her clientele includes Jennifer Lopez, Kate Moss, and Cindy Crawford. She is author of *The Ciminelli Solution: A Seven Day Plan for Radiant Skin*. She offers the most innovative signature skincare treatments using only the finest natural ingredients from the earth and oceans to nourish and detoxify your skin. Each service and product helps to bring your body back into balance, creating an inner peace and harmony that is the source of "The Ciminelli Glow."

Cross, Joe

www.RebootWithJoe.com
Joe Cross is a filmmaker, entrepreneur, author, and wellness advocate. He directed, produced, and was the subject of the award-winning documentary *Fat, Sick & Nearly Dead*; authored the *New York Times* bestseller *The Reboot with Joe Juice Diet*, which has been released globally in multiple languages; and is credited with having accelerated the plant-based eating and juicing movement

by media outlets including the *Wall Street Journal*, *The Times* of London, and *The Dr. Oz Show*. His website www.rebootwithjoe.com has become an integral meeting place for a community of more than 1 million Rebooters worldwide. His second documentary film, *Fat, Sick & Nearly Dead 2*, focuses on how to stay healthy in an unhealthy world. His third documentary is *The Kids Menu*. In the film, Joe meets with experts, parents, teachers, and kids, coming to the realization that childhood obesity isn't the real issue, but rather a symptom of bigger problems: The lack of knowledge of what healthy foods are. Lack of access to healthy and affordable options. And the influence of negative role models, whether a parent, teacher, or even a celebrity. In the film we see amazing programs in action, inspiring individuals paving the way for change, but most of all—kids, taking the lead in getting healthier options on their own menu.

Danoff, Dudley

www.TowerUrology.com
Dudley Danoff MD, FACS, is a male sexual health expert and founder of the Cedars-Sinai Medical Centre Tower Urology Group in Los Angeles, with thirty years' experience as a urologist. He is also the author of *The Ultimate Guide to Male Sexual Health*.

DePree, Barb

www.MiddleSexMD.com
Barb DePree, MD, has thirty years' experience as a gynecologist and women's health provider, and ten as a menopause care specialist. Her site offers advice and help for women who want to stay sexually active their whole lives. In her "Products" section she offers tastefully presented sex tools and sex enhancing devices with explanations about how they work and why she chose these items. She is also author of *Yes, You Can*, a "vaginal maintenance plan" to avoid unwanted changes in the "vaginal architecture."

Donsky, Andrea

www.andreadonsky.com
Andrea is a pioneer and visionary in the Natural Health Industry. She has combined her expertise as a Registered Holistic Nutritionist (RHN) and an entrepreneur to educate the public on living a healthy lifestyle. Andrea inspires people to make enlightened choices for healthy living through her businesses, books, articles, videos, speeches, and TV and radio appearances. Andrea founded Naturally Savvy in 2007, a website with unique content dedicated to healthy living from a holistic perspective. Among her numerous publications, Andrea co-authored *Unjunk Your Junk Food*, published by Simon and Schuster, a book that journalist, author, and mother Maria Shriver endorsed: "*Unjunk Your Junk Food* has certainly made me more aware about the food that my children eat and the effects it has on our body and mind." Andrea also co-authored two ebooks titled *Label Lessons: Your Guide to a Healthy Shopping Cart,* and *Label Lessons: Unjunk Your Kid's Lunch Box.* Andrea is the proud mother of three children who love seaweed, fish oil, and kale chips.

Ewers, Keesha

www.DrKeesha.com
Keesha Ewers, MD, is an integrative medicine expert, doctor of sexology, psychotherapist, and the founder and medical director of the Academy for Integrative Medicine Health Coach

Certification Program. Dr. Keesha has been in the medical field for more than 30 years. After being diagnosed with rheumatoid arthritis—an incurable disease according to Western medicine—she discovered how to reverse autoimmunity using her Freedom Framework® Method, which she has now used with thousands of her own patients and teaches to her health coach students in her online certification program. Dr. Keesha is a popular speaker, and the bestselling author of *Solving the Autoimmune Puzzle: The Woman's Guide to Reclaiming Emotional Freedom* and *Vibrant Health and Your Libido Story: A workbook for women who want to find, fix, and free their sexual desire.* You can listen to her *Healthy YOU!* radio show and find her programs at *DrKeesha.com*.

Fenster, Michael

www.chefdrmike.com
Michael S. Fenster, MD, FACC, FSCA & PEMBA, known to friends and fans simply as "Chef Dr. Mike," is *The Food Shaman.* He is a board-certified interventional cardiologist and professional chef. He currently holds faculty cross-appointments at The University of Montana College of Health Professions and Biomedical Sciences as well as The University of Montana Missoula College Culinary Arts Program. In addition to his clinical practice, he hosts a sponsored weekly show, *Journeys into Quantum Food*, available on iTunes. Chef Dr. Mike has appeared as an expert guest on many national radio and television programs, including *The Doctors* and *Fox National News.* He currently writes a regular column for *Psychology Today* and has authored several books including *The Fallacy of The Calorie: Why the Modern Western Diet Is Killing Us and How to Stop It* (Koehler Books, 2014), *Ancient Eats: The Greeks and Vikings* (Koehler Books, 2016), and *Food Shaman: The Art of Quantum Food* (Post Hill Press, June 2018), his latest offering. He was recently asked to be on the editorial board of the academic journal, *The Journal of Integrative Cardiology.*

Fleischmann, Nicole

www.AUCofNY.com
Nicole Fleischmann, MD, is the latest member to join AUCNY—White Plains Maple Avenue. She graduated summa cum laude from Downstate Medical Center in Brooklyn and completed her residency in Urology at Albert Einstein College of Medicine. She then pursued fellowship training at NYU Medical Center in female urology and voiding dysfunction. After one year as the Director of Female Urology and Pelvic Medicine at Mount Sinai Hospital in New York City she joined the practice in White Plains. Dr. Fleischmann's clinical interest and expertise is urinary incontinence and pelvic floor prolapse. She developed the urinary continence center specializing in both male and female urinary leakage. With state-of-the-art urodynamic testing, she diagnoses and treats complex issues in incontinence. She offers the laser treatment MonaLisa Touch®.

Frates, Beth

www.wellness-synergy.com
Beth Frates, MD, is a graduate of Harvard College and Stanford University School of Medicine. She completed her internship in medicine at Massachusetts General Hospital and went on to complete her residency in physical medicine and rehabilitation at the Harvard Medical School Program where she served as Chief Resident. She is currently an assistant clinical professor at

Harvard Medical School. Beth's passion for teaching has been recognized by Harvard Medical School where she has won several Excellence in Teaching Awards for her work in multiple pre-clinical courses, including The Human Central Nervous System and Behavior, Musculoskeletal System, Nutrition, and Introduction to the Profession. In the fall of 2014, she was invited to teach a course on Lifestyle Medicine which she created and delivered at the Harvard Extension School.

Gioffre, Daryl

www.getoffyouracid.com

Daryl Gioffre, DC, is a celebrity nutritionist and longevity expert who specializes in the alkaline diet. A former sugar addict turned health machine, Dr. Gioffre knows firsthand what it takes to overcome adversity and challenges in your health. His specialty is uncovering the root causes of inflammation and chronic illness (ACID!), using a comprehensive, yet simple, seven-step plan to make healthy changes more convenient and sustainable. The founder of the Gioffre Chiropractic Wellness Center and Alkamind, he is a board-certified chiropractor in the state of New York. He is the author of *Get Off Your Acid*: *7 Steps in 7 Days to Lose Weight, Fight Inflammation, and Reclaim Your Health & Energy*, published by the Hachette Book Group (division of Dacapo).

Hillhouse, Jill

www.jillhillhouse.com

Jill Hillhouse, BA, BPHE, CNP, RNT, is the author of *The Paleo Diabetes Diet Solution* as well as the bestselling book *The Best Baby Food*. She also writes articles for a number of national print and online publications. Jill is a passionate advocate of whole foods eating and nutrition education. She believes that health starts on your dinner plate and she uses diet and lifestyle shifts to mitigate and reverse health conditions. Jill focuses on addressing her clients' metabolic individuality as a key factor in her functional nutrition protocols and health coaching. A strong voice for self-advocacy, Jill encourages and empowers her clients to be active participants in their own health care. Working as a practitioner since 2001, Jill is part of the integrative health team at P3 Health Clinic in Toronto, Canada. She is also a Trusted Advisor for Zwell.ca, and a PRO with League.com. Jill is a Certified Nutritional Practitioner (CNP) from The Institute of Holistic Nutrition and has earned her Bachelor of Physical and Health Education (BPHE) and her BA in Psychology at Queen's University.

Irby, Susan

http://thebikinichef.com/product/food-healing-nutrition-program/

Susan Irby, CFNS, creator of the successful brand The Bikini Chef®, is one of the nation's foremost experts in fitness nutrition and recipe development, an accomplished public speaker, and media personality. Her seventeen years in the culinary industry, the past fourteen in health, fitness, and wellness, have earned Susan recognition as the leading lifestyle wellness and weight loss expert. Through her trademark 3-prong approach, Susan empowers others to sustain life-long health and weight management through her practical, no-fail approach to spiritual health, nutrition, and an active lifestyle. Susan is author of nine recipe and wellness books including *Substitute Yourself Skinny*, ranked twice by FOXNews.com in the Top 10 Best Diet Books, and

The Complete Idiot's Guide to Quinoa Cookbook. Susan's books and recipes have been featured in prestigious media outlets such as *FIRST for Women*, *Self*, *The New York Post*, and numerous other media outlets both in the US and internationally acclaimed outlets such as *The Mail on Sunday* and *BBC Radio*.

Kahn, Joel

www.drjoelkahn.com

Joel Kahn, MD, believes at his core that plant-based nutrition is the most powerful source of preventative medicine on the planet. Having practiced traditional cardiology since 1983, it was only after his own commitment to a plant-based vegan diet that he truly began to delve into the realm of non-traditional diagnostic tools, prevention tactics, and nutrition-based recovery protocols. These ideologies led him to change his approach and focus on being a holistic cardiologist. He passionately lectures throughout the country about the health benefits of a plant-based anti-aging diet inspiring a new generation of thought leaders to think scientifically and critically about the body's ability to heal itself through proper nutrition.

Kapoor, Deepak

www.AUCofNY.com

Deepak Kapoor, MD, is one of the youngest physicians to have been certified by the American Board of Urology. Dr. Kapoor is president of the Large Urology Group Practice Association, chairman of Access to Integrated Cancer Care, and founder and former president of the Integrated Medical Foundation.

Klaper, Michael

www.DoctorKlaper.com

Michael Klaper, MD, is a gifted clinician, internationally recognized teacher, and sought-after speaker on diet and health. He has practiced medicine for more than 40 years and is a leading educator in applied plant-based nutrition and integrative medicine. He is also the author of a successful book on cholesterol-free nutrition and an upcoming title (to be announced in 2018), as well as numerous DVDs and Videos on Demand, a series of "Healthy YOU Webinars," and dozens of articles. A source of inspiration advocating plant-based diets and the end of animal cruelty worldwide, Dr. Klaper contributed to the making of two PBS television programs: *Food for Thought* and the award-winning *Diet for a New America* movie based on the book of the same name.

Kroll, Mark

www.TheHypnosisExperience.com

Mark Kroll, BA, CH, received his BA in Psychology from the University of California at Santa Barbara, where he was part of the Call-Line (Community Assistance Listening Line) for three years. From 2001—2004, he was the Alcohol and Drug Abuse Family Specialist at the Army Substance Abuse Program at Schofield Barracks, Oahu, Hawaii. In 2006, he and his business partner launched The Hypnosis Experience.

The Hypnosis Experience has a simple mission: Provide quality, safe, family/corporate-friendly hypnotic services in areas of personal growth and well-being. Hypnosis is used to help clients achieve their behavioral goals including smoking cessation, improving study habits, overcoming phobias, relieving insomnia, and weight loss for both individuals and groups. Visit online and enjoy entertainment and self-help videos and downloads.

Liebman, Hollis

www.holliswashere.com
Hollis Lance Liebman has won national bodybuilding competitions, trained celebrities like Hugh Jackman and Jane Lynch, and worked as a fitness magazine editor and photographer. He has published twelve books on exercise and anatomy. He lives in Los Angeles, California. His latest books are *1,500 Stretches: The Complete Guide to Flexibility and Movement* and *Complete Physique: Your Ultimate Body Transformation.*

Macdonald, Erin

www.URockGirl.com
Erin Macdonald, RDN, has been a registered dietitian for twenty-three years. She is the co-founder of *U Rock Girl!* a health and wellness website for women, providing information, recipes, products, and services to nourish the mind, body, and spirit. Erin is the co-author of *No Excuses! 50 Healthy Ways to ROCK Breakfast!,* the first published cookbook for U Rock Girl, featuring nutritious and delicious breakfast recipes that will prevent the excuse, "I can't eat breakfast because..." She is also the co-author of *No Excuses! 50 Healthy Ways to ROCK Lunch and Dinner.* Erin sits on the Health Advisory Board of *Clean Eating Magazine* and co-writes a regular column, called "Ask the Dietitians." She also writes for *Oxygen Magazine* and ACE Fitness, and has also been quoted in numerous magazines and online articles. Erin has appeared on radio, television, and DVDs discussing various hot topics regarding nutrition, weight, and wellness. She has presented many lectures focusing on weight management, heart-healthy cooking, sports nutrition, blood sugar health, and pediatric nutrition, and writes a blog on health, nutrition, fitness, wellness, and motivation on www.URockGirl.com. Passionate about cooking and recipe development, Erin teaches monthly cooking classes featuring original clean-eating recipes.

Manning, Drew

www.Fit2Fat2Fit.com
Drew Manning is the NY Times best-selling author of the book, *Fit2Fat2Fit,* and is best known for his Fit2Fat2Fit.com experiment that went viral online. He's been featured on shows like *Dr. Oz, Good Morning America, The View* and many more. His experiment has since become a hit TV show, called *Fit to Fat to Fit,* airing on A&E and Lifetime. Drew also has a very successful podcast called The Fit2Fat2Fit Experience and has recently reached over 1 million downloads. Since his self-experiment went viral, Drew has helped thousands of people learn to live a healthy lifestyle and completely transform their lives.

Marin, Vanessa

www.vmtherapy.com

Vanessa Marin, MA, is a licensed psychotherapist, coach, and writer who helps people stop feeling embarrassed and start having more fun in the bedroom. She studied human sexuality at Brown University and has been featured in publications like the *New York Times*, *Real Simple*, CNN, *O, The Oprah Magazine*, and *The Times*. Whether in her work coaching clients one-on-one via email and video chat, or through her online sex education programs like *The Modern Man's Guide to Conquering Performance Pressure* and *Finishing School: Learn How To Orgasm*, she finds immense joy in helping people discover (or rediscover!) their spark.

Masley, Steven

www.DrMasley.com

Steven Masley, MD, is a physician, nutritionist, trained chef, author, and the creator of the #1 health program for public television, *30 Days to a Younger Heart*. He helps motivated people tune up their brain, heart, and sexual performance. He is a fellow with three prestigious organizations: the American Heart Association, American College of Nutrition, and American Academy of Family Physicians. His research focuses on the impact of lifestyle choices on brain function, heart disease, and aging. His passion is empowering people to achieve optimal health through comprehensive assessments and lifestyle changes.

As a best-selling author, he has published several books: *Ten Years Younger, The 30-Day Heart Tune-Up, Smart Fat*, and his latest book, *The Better Brain Solution*, plus numerous scientific articles. His work has been viewed by millions on PBS, the Discovery Channel, *The Today Show*, and over 500 media interviews. He also completed a chef internship at the Four Seasons Restaurant in Seattle, WA, and he has performed cooking demonstrations at Cal-a-Vie Health Spa, Canyon Ranch, the Pritikin Longevity Center, and for multiple television appearances. As a speaker during his career, Dr. Masley has spoken for over 300 physician continuing medical education (CME) events, and for over 700 public presentations on a variety of topics related to health, cognitive function, aging, and cardiovascular disease. He continues to see patients and publish research from his medical clinic in St. Petersburg, Florida.

Masters, Tess

www.TheBlenderGirl.com

Tess Masters is an actress, cook, lifestyle personality, and author of *The Blender Girl, The Perfect Blend, The Detox Dynamo Cleanse*, and *The Blender Girl Smoothies* app and book. She shares her enthusiasm for healthy living at theblendergirl.com. As a spokesperson, presenter, and recipe developer, Tess collaborates with leading food and lifestyle brands. She and her healthy fast food have been featured in the *LA Times, Washington Post, InStyle, Real Simple, Prevention, Family Circle, Vegetarian Times, FoodNetwork.com, Shape.com, Glamour.com, Yahoo.com*, and *Parents. com*, among other publications around the world.

Mattocks, Charles

www.charlesmattocks.com/reversed

Celebrity chef Charles Mattocks, also known as the Poor Chef, nephew to the late reggae legend Bob Marley, has created a show to change the health and medical industry forever. He is an award-winning film producer, as well as an international diabetes advocate, IDF Blue Circle Champion, and American Diabetes Association published author. Charles made a name for himself on such shows as CNN, *Dr. Oz* and *The Today Show*. As a best-selling author and spokesperson, Charles was on the road to becoming a household name when he was diagnosed with Type II diabetes, only 4 years ago. After such devastating news Charles started a global mission for not only his life, but also for the millions struggling with diabetes. *Reversed* was born out of a desire to help, inspire, and educate billions worldwide. Charles created a movement, now a first-ever reality TV show, as a blueprint for not only tackling diabetes, but many other illnesses as well, while improving health. In this show, five people from all over the world are followed in a house for seven days to do 'REVERSED,' changing the way they eat, drink, think, exercise, and live healthy with diabetes.

McDermott, Denise

www.drdenisemd.com

Denise McDermott, MD, has been in private practice in Southern California since 2001. She completed her adult psychiatry residency at Emory University in Atlanta, Georgia, and her child psychiatry residency at UCLA. As a medical doctor with board certifications in both adult and child psychiatry, she treats children, adolescents, and adults. Her goal is to empower people to live the best life possible. Her approach is to encourage people to believe in wellness, not illness, and to lead a balanced, healthy lifestyle. Dr. Denise utilizes a multidisciplinary approach to medicine, where she integrates her Western medicine psychiatric training using the Bio/Psycho/Social framework coupled with a Spirit/Mind/Body approach for mental health treatment of the whole person. In 2016, she started her podcast *The Dr. Denise Show*, and she released her ebook, *Mental Health and How to Thrive* in the fall of that year.

McElfish, Wendy K.

www.wendykathleenphotography.com
www.instagram.com/wendykathleenphotography/

Wendy McElfish is a free spirit photographer and teacher. She did the 2nd edition of Erin Macdonald's breakfast book *No Excuses! 50 Healthy Ways to ROCK Breakfast!* She also did the photography for *No Excuses! 50 Healthy Ways to ROCK Lunch and Dinner!*

Miller, Robin

www.WellHealed.net
www.TriuneMed.com

Robin Miller, MD, MHS, is an integrative medical doctor and proponent of the connection between health and happiness, an advocate of dancing, and co-author of *Healed! Health & Wellness for the 21st Century: Wisdom, Secrets, and Fun Straight from the Leading Edge.* She is also author of *The Smart Woman's Guide to Midlife and Beyond* and *Kids Ask the Doctor.*

Moretti, Heidi

www.dietdetectiverd.com

Heidi Moretti, MS, RD, LN, is a nutritionist, nutrition researcher, and virtual dietitian. Her passion for integrative and functional medicine is "at the core of her being." She has practiced in a hospital setting for eighteen years. She finds energy and joy from helping people on the path to recovery. Being a nutrition researcher gave Heidi a deep understanding of what makes up good research versus hype or fuel for media propaganda. Heidi became a virtual dietitian to dive deeper to help people find root causes to their illnesses and help people in ways that conventional medicine can't fully address. Heidi has seen firsthand that the foods we eat, including herbs and key amounts of nutrients, are life-changing. She says, "Health is not the absence of disease, it is the presence of vitality!"

Nunez, Michelle

http://www.medskinboutique.com

Michelle Nunez, a Master Esthetician, has been in the skincare industry for more than seven years. She is a graduate of the 1,200-hour Master Esthetics program from Catherine Hinds Institute of Esthetics. Her certifications include microdermabrasion, dermaplaning, chemical peels, Environ facials, Rezenerate facial, lash lift, brow/lash tinting, and cryoclear.

Panasevich, Jake

www.YogaWithJake.com

Jake Panasevich is a yoga and wellness mentor and teacher to large, committed groups of beginners and advanced students alike. With a strong wrestling, coaching, and writing background, Jake developed "Yoga for Dudes." Jake inspires students to get committed, get stronger, and learn to love life and flourish in it. Drawing from over seven intensive trainings, Jake threads the most beneficial practices from different modalities into a unique yoga experience for inflexible, stressed, overworked, regular Americans.

Paul, Margaret

www.innerbonding.com

Margaret Paul, PhD, is the co-creator of Inner Bonding® and author/co-author of several best-selling books, including *Do I Have to Give Up Me to Be Loved by You?*, *Inner Bonding*, *Healing Your Aloneness*, *The Healing Your Aloneness Workbook*, *Do I Have to Give Up Me to Be Loved by My Kids?*, and *Do I Have to Give Up Me to Be Loved by God?* Her books have been distributed around the world and have been translated into eleven languages. Margaret holds a PhD in psychology and is a relationship expert, noted public speaker, workshop leader, educator, chaplain, consultant, and artist. She has appeared on many radio and TV shows, including *Oprah*. She has successfully worked with thousands of individuals, couples, and business relationships and taught classes and seminars since 1967. Margaret continues to work with individuals and couples throughout the world and offers phone and Skype sessions. Her new book is *Diet for Divine Connection*.

Petrucci, Kellyann

www.DrKellyann.com

Kellyann Petrucci, MS, ND, is a holistic weight-loss and health specialist and author of *Dr. Kellyann's 21-Day Bone Broth Diet*. She promotes bone broth for a slimmer, younger you. Dr. Kellyann came to realize the ancient power of collagen and bone broth to heal the gut and to slow aging while studying biological medicine at the Marion Foundation and Paracelsus Klinik, Switzerland. By focusing her practice on a lifestyle that stops and reverses inflammation, Dr. Kellyann is able to help patients and readers reduce dangerous belly fat to become slimmer, younger, and healthier.

Pollock, David

www.justaskdavid.com

Named one of the "20 to Know" by *Global Cosmetics Industry*, David Pollock has developed top-selling items for some of the most prestigious names in beauty—including Bliss, Smashbox, Lancôme, L'Oreal, and many more. After spending two decades creating some of the most recognized products in the industry, David chose to make a dramatic shift in his professional life to focus on Safe Beauty. He was inspired to take this leap after assisting several loved ones through their battles with cancer. He is a published author, a frequent keynote speaker, and a producer and co-host of the weekly podcast *Just Ask David*, which hit the #1 spot on iTunes in the fashion and beauty category within one month of its launch. Today, David advises a number of different skin-care brands and retailers, and is a consumer advocate, empowering people to take control of their health and beauty—from the inside out. His Florida-based company, Brand Labs USA, LLC, produces science-based, high-performance beauty products for a number of recognized brands and follows strict guidelines for Safe Beauty. Nothing produced at the facility contains harsh chemicals, parabens, PEGs, glycols, sulfates, petrochemicals, synthetic fragrances, or artificial dyes.

Ramirez, Marc

www.ChickpeaAndBean.com

Marc Ramirez and his wife Kim started a non-profit after Marc's almost miraculous recovery from a long list of ailments that nearly killed him, including erectile dysfunction. Called Chickpea and Bean (Kim is Chickpea and Marc is Bean), the nonprofit's mission is to educate people about the power and benefits of a whole food, plant-based lifestyle.

Ramsey, Debbie

www.MusicAndDance.com

www.CarolinaDanceClub.com

Debbie Ramsey has been dancing since she was two and a half years old and is a mega award-winning swing dancer, master dance instructor, contest judge, and choreographer for both movies and television. She has been a dance coach to actors Donald Sutherland, Brendan Fraser,

Sylvester Stallone, and Dolly Parton. Her film and television dance credits include lead dancer with Donald Sutherland in *Younger and Younger*, dance work on *Back to the Future 1 & 2*, *Fast Times at Ridgemont High*, *Hill Street Blues*, *Murder She Wrote*, *Simon & Simon*, *The Fall Guy*, and *Major Dad*.

Shemek, Lori

https://drlorishemek.com/

Lori Shemek, PhD, CNC, is a nutrition and weight loss expert, a best-selling author, and specialist in weight loss resistance. She is well known as a pioneer in creating global awareness of low-level inflammation and how it is responsible for and the core cause of most illness, disease, faster aging and weight gain. Also known as "The Inflammation Terminator," she had been sending out the message about inflammation long before it became a buzzword. Dr. Shemek has uncovered the pathway to the core cause of excess weight: inflamed fat cells that not only promote unwanted excess weight gain and belly fat, but poor health as well. She shows people how to spot sneaky foods that create weight gain, kick sugar addiction to the curb, and shift from eating the wrong foods to foods that burn fat. Dr. Shemek is the author of *How to Fight FATflammation!* and the best-selling author of *Fire-Up Your Fat Burn!*

Simon, Julie M.

http://www.overeatingrecovery.com

Julie M. Simon is a licensed psychotherapist and life coach with a full-time private practice specializing in eating and body image challenges and associated mood disturbances such as depression and anxiety. In addition to her specialty, she provides psychotherapy and life coaching services for a variety of other issues. She holds a master's degree in clinical psychology from Antioch University, Los Angeles. In addition to her education and more than twenty-seven years of experience as a psychotherapist, she is a certified personal trainer with twenty-five years of experience designing personalized exercise and nutrition programs for various populations. Julie created the Twelve-Week Emotional Eating Recovery Coaching Program, which has been running for more than twenty-five years.

Spiker, Ted

www.tedspiker.com

Ted Spiker, MS, is the chair of the department of journalism at the University of Florida. He teaches advanced magazine writing and sports media & society, as well as other magazine and writing courses. Spiker, who was an editor at *Men's Health* before coming to UF, has had hundreds of stories published (primarily about health and fitness) in TIME.com, Esquire.com, Outside; *O: The Oprah Magazine, Women's Health, Runner's World, Fortune*, and many other magazines and digital platforms.

Spiker writes the "Big Guy Blog" for RunnersWorld.com, has co-authored about twenty books, and authored one. He was once named by Greatist.com as one of the 100 most influential people in health and fitness. He was named the 2016–17 Teacher of the Year at the University of Florida.

Stobo, Diana

www.DianaStobo.com

www.TheSpaCostaRica.com

Over the past fifteen years Diana Stobo has written more than fifteen books, including the two-time award-winning *Get Naked Fast - A guide to stripping away the foods that weigh you down*, and has spoken around the world on health and wellness. Stobo also has coached thousands of people back to good health and created many products in the health and wellness category. Currently, her biggest passion is her hotel, *The Retreat Costa Rica*, a lifestyle hotel that opened May 2014 and has already been dubbed "Best Wellness Spa in the Americas" by World Boutique Awards and #1 Detox Spa Worldwide by *W* magazine. Diana also created and formulated *The Truth Bar*, a completely innovative probiotic/prebiotic bar that is available in stores across the US.

Her specialty has always been food as a modality for change, understanding the true nature of the anatomy and its metaphysical connections. But her education and expertise lie in life transformation and spirit coaching, through quantum physics and the law of attraction.

Currently, Diana is venturing into Wellness Community Real Estate as well as expanding The Retreat Costa Rica and the Truth Bar line of functional snack bars. She is the co-founder and chief formulator of *Truth Bar* and the founder and CEO of *The Retreat Costa Rica* and Diana Stobo, LLC.

Stosny, Steven

www.compassionpower.com

Steven Stosny, PhD, is the founder of Compassion*Power*. A renowned author and media consultant on relationships, anger, and abuse, Dr. Stosny grew up in a violent home. He learned the healing power of compassion from his abused mother.

Dr. Stosny has appeared on many TV and radio shows, including several guest appearances on the Oprah Winfrey Show. He has been the subject of interviews in national newspapers and magazines, including the *New York Times*, *Wall Street Journal*, and *USA Today*. He is the co-author of *Get Naked Fast: A Guide to Stripping Away the Foods That Weigh You Down*.

Vij, Pankaj

http://doctorvij.com

Pankaj Vij, MD, FACP, author of *Turbo Metabolism*, is passionate about nutrition, fitness, and human performance. He has been on a quest to help people slow down the aging process and optimize human performance, thereby enhancing health span, not just life span. He practices what he preaches by following a low-glycemic, anti-inflammatory, real food diet, and engaging in regular physical activity, meditation, and sleep. He adds music and humor for good measure. Board certified in internal medicine and obesity medicine, Dr. Vij has been practicing medicine since 1997. He has helped thousands of people achieve and maintain their goal weight and improve their fitness level, thus helping them live healthier and longer with fewer medications.

Weiner-Davis, Michele

www.DivorceBusting.com

Michele Weiner-Davis, MSW, is an internationally renowned relationship expert, best-selling author, marriage therapist, and professional speaker. Among the first in her field to courageously speak out about the pitfalls of unnecessary divorce, Michele has been active in spearheading the now-popular movement urging couples to make their marriages work and keep their families together. Michele is the director of The Divorce Busting® Center and the founder of www .divorcebusting.com. She has been a frequent guest on shows such as *Oprah, 20/20, 48 Hours, The TODAY show, Good Morning America, CBS Evening News*, and so on. Her work as been featured in many major newspapers and magazines.

Wider, Jennifer

http://drwider.com

Jennifer Wider, MD, is a nationally renowned women's health expert, author, and radio host. She has appeared on *The Today Show, CBS News, ABC News Nightline, Fox News, Good Day NY, HuffPost Live*, and *The Bethenny Show*. Dr. Wider is a medical adviser to *Cosmopolitan* magazine and hosts a weekly radio segment on Sirius XM Stars called "Am I Normal?" She has been heard on Bloomberg Radio, Howard Stern, Oprah Radio, WABC-AM Talk Radio, among many other stations across the country. Dr. Wider is the author of four books: *The Savvy Woman Patient, The Doctor's Complete College Girls' Health Guide, The New Mom's Survival Guide* and *Got Teens? The Doctor Moms' Guide to Sexuality, Social Media and other Adolescent Realities* with Dr. Logan Levkoff.

Wildflower, Joy

Joy Wildflower, MS, PE, is a registered Professional Engineer and has worked for the California State Drinking Water Program since 2005. Along with ensuring public water systems serve clean, potable water, she has assisted public water systems through fires, floods, and drought.

ORGANIZATIONS

Carolina Dance Club

www.MusicAndDance.com

www.CarolinaDanceClub.com

Debbie Ramsey and Wesley Boz are known for their dance awards in the West Coast Swing Dancing community and choreography work on television. They own Music and Dance Productions, a DJ company offering party packages and dance instruction.

Carolina Dance Club is headquartered in Raleigh, North Carolina, but has a national reach; Debbie Ramsey works tirelessly in the swing dance community nationwide.

Environmental Protection Agency (EPA)

www.EPA.gov

Search here for more information on endocrine disruption and endocrine disrupting chemicals (EDCs) and drinking water.

Environmental Working Group (EWG)

www.EWG.org

EWG publishes the yearly Clean Fifteen and the Dirty Dozen, a list of the top clean (least amount of pesticide residue) and dirty (highest amount of pesticide residue) foods. They also list genetically modified produce and look at water issues.

Men's Health

www.MensHealth.com

Publisher of *Men's Health* magazine and devoted to all aspects of health, healing, and happiness for men.

North American Menopause Society (NAMS)

www.Menopause.org

North America's leading nonprofit organization dedicated to promoting the health and quality of life of all women during midlife and beyond through an understanding of menopause and healthy aging.

USA Dance

www.USADance.org

This national group has local chapters in most US cities and states. Their goal is to improve the quality and quantity of ballroom dancing in the United States. Their website provides links and locations to local USA Dance groups. Most USA Dance groups hold dances once a month, but they are also great source for local dance studios that offer lessons and other dance groups that meet locally.

PRODUCTS

Al Dente Gluten Free Pasta

www.aldentepasta.com
Gluten Free Pastas made with white bean and brown rice flour, making it high in protein and rich in fiber.

Avohass Avocado Oil

www.Avohass.com
Organic avocado oil.

Coconut Bliss

www.CoconutBliss.com
Creamy, dairy-free frozen desserts, including ice cream.

Bone Broth

www.drkellyannstore.com
This warm, luscious broth will satisfy you down to your toes. It's flavored with onions, parsley, and garlic and simmered for twenty-four hours with a touch of vinegar to draw even more nutrients out of the bone.

Devil's Envy Spice

www.DevilsEnvySpice.com
Handcrafted Mexican spice

Essential Oils

https://www.dietdetectiverd.com
Essential oils can be used to support a variety of health conditions, from diabetes and arthritis to digestive issues and skin conditions.

Modern Table Meals

www.moderntable.com
Pastas made from a blend of lentils, rice, and pea protein.

MonaLisa Touch®

www.MonaLisaTouch.com
A laser treatment aimed at reversing the effects of vaginal atrophy.

Prenatal Yoga-Shiva Rea

www.shivarea.com
Shiva Rea offers a wide variety of yoga online.

Sex Toys

www.amazon.com or find your favorite sex toy shop in person or online

Sexual Stimulation Devices for Women and Their Partners

www.MiddleSexMD.com
Look in the products section for products tested and recommended by Dr. Barb DePree and her staff. Each one is described in detail with one or more photographs, and includes instructions on why they recommend the device, how it works, and how to use it.

Skin-care products

www.justaskdavid.com
www.susanciminelli.com
These are the products I use for all my skin-care needs.

Woo for Play

www.wooforplay.com
All-natural and organic personal lubricant

Youtrients

www.youtrients.me
"We are able to make personalized supplements for every single customer based on their unique genes using the best materials on the planet. This is Youtrients™."

CONVERSION CHARTS

METRIC AND IMPERIAL CONVERSIONS
(These conversions are rounded for convenience)

Ingredient	Cups/Tablespoons/Teaspoons	Ounces	Grams/Milliliters
Butter	1 cup/ 16 tablespoons/ 2 sticks	8 ounces	230 grams
Cheese, shredded	1 cup	4 ounces	110 grams
Cornstarch	1 tablespoon	0.3 ounce	8 grams
Cream cheese	1 tablespoon	0.5 ounce	14.5 grams
Flour, all-purpose	1 cup/1 tablespoon	4.5 ounces/0.3 ounce	125 grams/8 grams
Flour, whole wheat	1 cup	4 ounces	120 grams
Fruit, dried	1 cup	4 ounces	120 grams
Fruits or veggies, chopped	1 cup	5 to 7 ounces	145 to 200 grams
Fruits or veggies, puréed	1 cup	8.5 ounces	245 grams
Honey, maple syrup, or corn syrup	1 tablespoon	0.75 ounce	20 grams
Liquids: cream, milk, water, or juice	1 cup	8 fluid ounces	240 milliliters
Oats	1 cup	5.5 ounces	150 grams
Salt	1 teaspoon	0.2 ounces	6 grams
Spices: cinnamon, cloves, ginger, or nutmeg (ground)	1 teaspoon	0.2 ounce	5 milliliters
Sugar, brown, firmly packed	1 cup	7 ounces	200 grams
Sugar, white	1 cup/1 tablespoon	7 ounces/0.5 ounce	200 grams/12.5 grams
Vanilla extract	1 teaspoon	0.2 ounce	4 grams

OVEN TEMPERATURES

Fahrenheit	Celsius	Gas Mark
225°	110°	¼
250°	120°	½
275°	140°	1
300°	150°	2
325°	160°	3
350°	180°	4
375°	190°	5
400°	200°	6
425°	220°	7
450°	230°	8

INDEX

ACKNOWLEDGMENTS

My gratitude to Dr. Kellyann Petrucci for introducing me to my fantastic agent, Margot Hutchison. Dr. Petrucci instantly loved my book idea, and Margot has worked tirelessly to ensure this book became a reality.

Hats off to the creator of the delicious and healthy recipes, Erin Macdonald, RDN. I'm beyond thrilled and thankful for her work! I highly recommend you purchase her amazing books.

Wendy K. McElfish, our photographer, who was referred by Erin and whose images of the delicious recipes are mouth-watering!

Huge thanks to everyone at Skyhorse Publishing, especially my editor, Leah Zarra.

My career in radio and television has been boosted at every turn by the support and encouragement of three incredible women in the industry. Donna Gould was instrumental in getting my radio show "It's Your Health" on NPR, bringing my career to a whole new level. Becky Lauer and Rachel Kessler not only provide me with amazing guests for my shows, but are also helping with the promotion of this book. You gals rock!

No words can express how grateful I am for my amazing husband and the life we've built together. He's made so many sacrifices that allow me to go after my dreams. I love you, Hon! I also want to thank my wonderful daughter, who is the light of my life.

Thanks to my friends Chris Harvey, Michael Farca, Kevin Hammontree, and Chris Davis who were there for me while this book was forming in my mind and helped me bring it to life by sharing ideas and making me laugh!

Thanks to my father-in-law, David Davis, who lovingly spends time with his granddaughter every day—this book and my other on-air responsibilities would not materialize without you.

The biggest-ever thanks (beyond words) to my two awesome siblings for their undying support, for being marvelous, for co-writing this book, for staying up late and getting up early so we could span the six-hour time difference to hang out on Google Docs when we got tired of talking over each other on the phone, and for using "I" messages, even in the face of exhaustion. I love you both!

And to all of the experts listed in the book, who took time out of your busy lives, thank you. Your contributions are helping us all to help others be their best selves.